THIRD EDITION

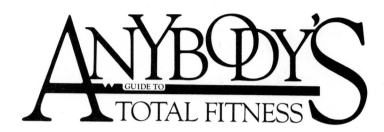
ANYBODY'S GUIDE TO TOTAL FITNESS

Len Kravitz, M.A.
San Jose State University

Designed and Illustrated By
Jill Pankey

Edited By
Susan Pate, Ph.D.

KENDALL/HUNT PUBLISHING COMPANY
2460 Kerper Boulevard P.O. Box 539 Dubuque, Iowa 52004-0539

Dedicated with love to my mom,
who has always believed in me.

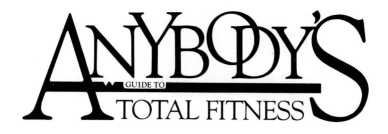

CONTENTS

EDITORIAL ADVISORY BOARD

ACKNOWLEDGMENTS

I would like to express my deep appreciation and gratitude to my editorial advisory board of Dr. Carol L. Christensen, Dr. Craig J. Cisar, Dr. Gail G. Evans, Dr. Susan Kutner, Lori Leeds, R.P.T., Dr. Thomas A. MacLean, Dr. Susan Pate, Dr. Robert Pearl, Dr. Jay D. Pruzansky, Dr. Norman T. Reynolds, Richard V. Schroeder, M.S. Dr. Phillip A. Sienna, and Dr. Robert J. Zick. Their advice, expertise, and thoughtful review of this book were invaluable.

I sincerely thank the following people who have made generous contributions to this project and deserve special acknowledgement: Molly Burke, Mert and Tanya Carpenter, Kim Drummond, Janice Earle, Carrie Ekins, Eric Finch. Dixie Fisher, Jerry Gonsalves, Jean Harding, Louise Herndon, Michael Le Doux, Shirley H. M. Reekie, Pauline Reimer, Joe Samuels, Wendy Russum, Dolores Sargent, Debbie Sporleder, Carol Sullivan, Pamela Staver, and Teri Wexted.

I would also like to thank the following special people who have been a source of inspiration and have guided me in countless ways: Covert Bailey, Dr. Barton Byers, Dr. Laurence Berkowitz, Ed and Shirley Burke, Don Callahan, Roy Cerrito, Retta Chavkin, Dr. Barbara Conry, Yvonne Cotton, Peter and Kathie Davis, Anita Del Grande, Jerry Dollard, Dr. Jacqueline Douglass, Ronda Gates, Dr. Telemachos A. Greanias, Dr. William F. Gustafson, C. Lansing Hays, Ellen Herbst, Dr. Vivian H. Heyward, Dr. Clair W. Jennett, DeAun Kizer, Bob Kravitz, Joyce Malone, Frank Napier, Dr. Bruce Ogilvie, Lawrence R. Petulla, Doug Sporleder, Marty Urand, and Neil Wiley.

For their enthusiastic support, I am grateful to my friends at the Los Gatos Athletic Club, the faculty and staff of Human Performance at San Jose State University, and everyone at Aerobics Plus.

I am also deeply indebted to my friend Chuck Drummond for providing such wise counsel and friendship.

To Dr. Susan Pate, my editor and lifetime friend, I thank you in a thousand different ways.

To Jill Pankey, my illustrator, I thank you for your artistic imagination and for the many hours of hard work you devoted to this book to make it come to life.

INTRODUCTION

A HEALTHY WAY OF LIFE

Living and enjoying life to its fullest is a wonderful goal. And you can have it! Fitness is a way of life which allows you to function and perform at your best. It's a harmonic balance of prescribed exercise, healthy eating habits, preventative health care, effective stress management, and a common sense lifestyle. Your level of fitness helps determine the quality of your life. You are in control of how you look, feel, and live.

The following information is based on sound physiological principles and research. With a minimal investment of your time you can follow these concepts and create a fitness plan that will help you obtain the most out of your life.

I have presented a specific aerobics program for you. You may wish to supplement it with a running, swimming, or cycling program of your own.

Be patient, use your knowledge, set your goals, listen to your body, and commit yourself to a healthy way of life.

STARTING OUT

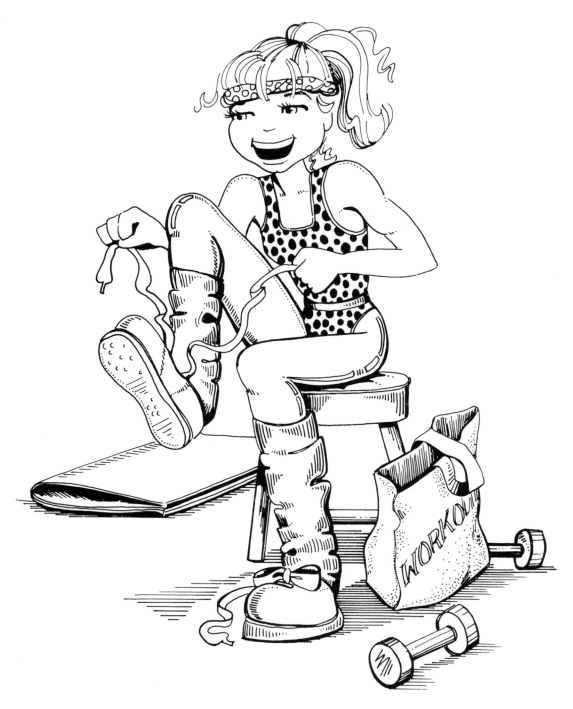

EXERCISE: WHAT IT WILL DO FOR YOU

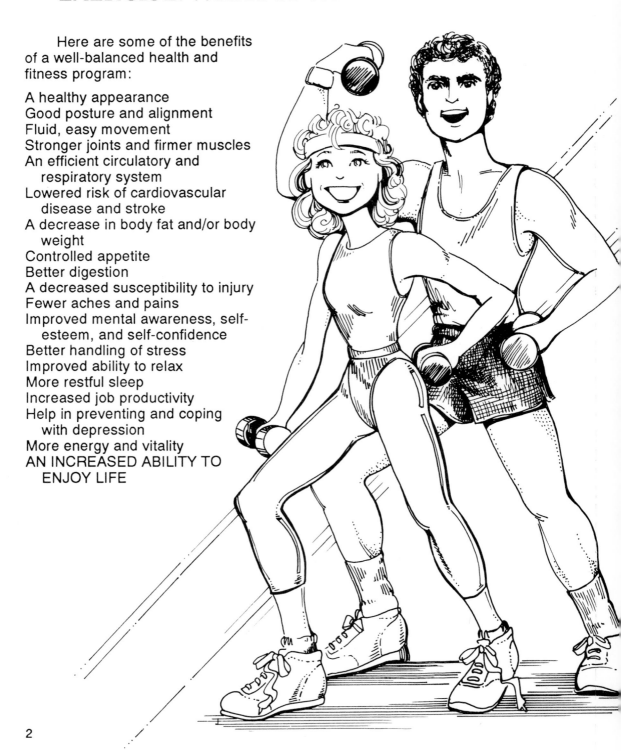

Here are some of the benefits of a well-balanced health and fitness program:

A healthy appearance
Good posture and alignment
Fluid, easy movement
Stronger joints and firmer muscles
An efficient circulatory and
 respiratory system
Lowered risk of cardiovascular
 disease and stroke
A decrease in body fat and/or body
 weight
Controlled appetite
Better digestion
A decreased susceptibility to injury
Fewer aches and pains
Improved mental awareness, self-
 esteem, and self-confidence
Better handling of stress
Improved ability to relax
More restful sleep
Increased job productivity
Help in preventing and coping
 with depression
More energy and vitality
AN INCREASED ABILITY TO
 ENJOY LIFE

STICKIN' TO IT!

10 RULES FOR EXERCISE SUCCESS

More than half of the people starting an exercise program drop out after six months. These tips will steer you towards success in exercise.

1. Write out a **health** and **fitness** evaluation list—what you do right (don't smoke, good eating habits, no substance abuse, etc.) and what you need to correct (lack of regular exercise, posture, high emotional stress, etc.). Then figure out what you can do to shift more entries to the "right" side.

2. Set realistic long- and short-term fitness goals. Write them down and solicit the support from someone close to you. Reward yourself as goals are achieved (a show, new outfit, a book, etc.).

3. Find a workout companion with a fitness level and goals similar to yours. Pick an exercise activity or class you both enjoy and **commit** to it!

4. Schedule your exercise three to five days per week. Choose a "special" time of day and be selfish about preserving that time for your body and general well-being.

5. Listen to your body and progress slowly in the beginning. Most injuries in fitness come from doing too much, too soon, too fast, and too hard. (Don't exercise if you are sick.)

6. Don't let early awkwardness or uneven skill development get you down (it happens to everyone). And try not to compare yourself to others.

7. Wear comfortable exercise clothing and proper shoes.

8. Plan your exercise at least two hours after a big meal or at least an hour before.

9. Be patient; exercise has many immediate and delayed benefits. Your time will come!

10. Be aware of the signs of overexertion: breathlessness, dizziness, tightness or pain in the chest, loss of muscle control, and nausea. If you experience any of these signs, stop immediately. See your physician to determine the cause.

3

THE KEY COMPONENTS OF FITNESS

Your body is a complex mechanism designed for action. Being physically fit means that the heart, blood vessels, lungs, and muscles function at optimal efficiency. Here are five key components of health-related physical fitness that you need to be concerned with:

1. **Cardiorespiratory Endurance/ Aerobic Conditioning** is the ability of the body's heart, lungs, blood vessels, and major muscle groups to persist in prolonged vigorous exercise such as brisk walking, jogging, swimming, aerobic dancing, rowing, cycling, rope skipping, skating, and cross-country skiing. Regular aerobic conditioning may prevent or reduce the likelihood of cardiovascular disease. Cardiorespiratory endurance is the most important component of physical fitness.

2. **Muscular Strength** is the ability of the muscles to exert maximal or near maximal force against resistance. Stronger muscles protect the joints they surround and reduce the incidence of injury from physical activity.

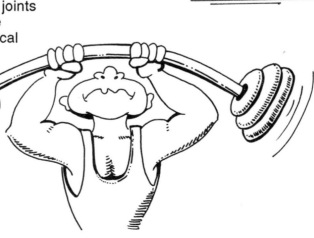

3. **Muscular Endurance** is the ability of skeletal muscle to exert force (not necessarily maximal) over an extended period of time. Strength, skill, performance, speed of movement, and power are closely associated with this component.

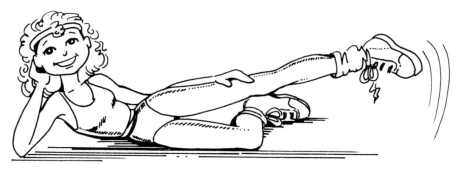

4. **Flexibility** is the range of motion of the muscles and joints of the body. It has to do with your skeletal muscles' natural and conditioned ability to extend beyond their normal resting length. Increased flexibility will enhance performance and reduce the incidence of injury.

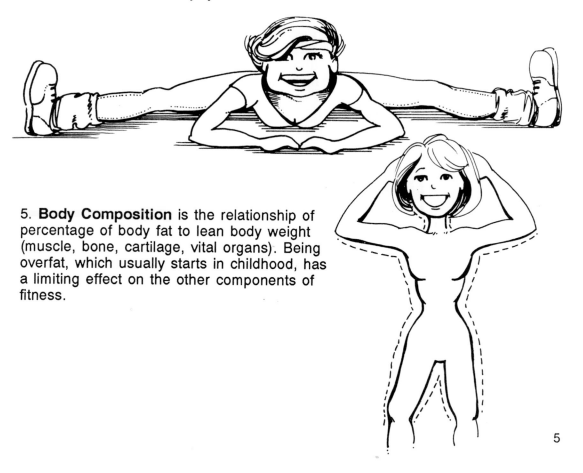

5. **Body Composition** is the relationship of percentage of body fat to lean body weight (muscle, bone, cartilage, vital organs). Being overfat, which usually starts in childhood, has a limiting effect on the other components of fitness.

ENERGY FOR EXERCISE

To exercise and do work for daily activities your body uses a chemical called ATP (adenosine triphosphate) like a car uses gasoline. ATP is produced by metabolizing the foods you eat, particularly carbohydrates and fats. Depending upon the intensity and duration of the activity, you produce ATP through either aerobic or anaerobic metabolism.

Aerobic (with oxygen) metabolism is the most efficient and main energy production system. This metabolic pathway cannot work unless there is sufficient oxygen available in the tissues during exercise. Prolonged vigorous activity over five minutes activates your aerobic metabolism; however, at least 20 minutes of this kind of activity is recommended to enhance your aerobic capacity.

Anaerobic (without oxygen) metabolism is utilized for situations requiring quick bursts of energy such as lifting weights, running short races, jumping, and throwing. Although less efficient than the aerobic system, it can quickly generate the ATP needed at the muscle site. Anaerobic metabolism may be called upon during aerobic conditioning if your intensity increases beyond the ability of your system to deliver oxygen (such as finishing a long run with a sprint or a section of high kicks during an aerobic program).

ON YOUR MARK, GET SET . . . WAIT!

It is always a good idea to undergo a medical examination before embarking on a strenuous program of exercise.

1. With your physician, write up a personal medical profile including a history of high blood pressure, chest pain, heart arrhythmia, or shortness of breath. Determine your coronary heart disease risk. Here's a list of heart disease risk factors and what you can do about them.

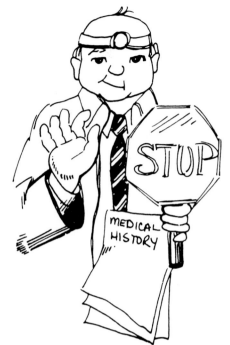

	RISK FACTOR	IMPROVED BY
A)	Age	(Not controllable)
B)	Sex	(Not controllable)
C)	Family history of heart disease	Although you are not able to alter your genetic make-up, new research suggests that physical activity can reduce this risk
D)	High blood pressure	Physical activity, weight
E)	Abnormal cholesterol levels	control, cessation of smoking, stress management, improved diet (less salt, fat, and red meat)
F)	Smoking	Stop smoking, alternative gratifying activities
G)	Obesity	Physical activity, weight control, improved diet (less animal fat, more unrefined carbohydrates), alternative gratifying activities
H)	Physical inactivity	Physical activity
I)	High blood sugar (or diabetes)	Physical activity, weight control, improved diet
J)	High emotional stress and tension	Physical activity, no smoking, relaxation techniques

2. Get a complete physical exam.
3. Upon completion of the exam, your physician will be able to recommend whether a stress test is warranted. This is an electrocardiographic record of your heart's rhythm and adaptability to stress, tested through graded exercise on a treadmill or stationary bicycle.

HOW FIT ARE YOU?

Here are some simple self-assessment tests to help determine or monitor your level of fitness. Periodically retest yourself to monitor your progress. Stop if you feel any nausea, discomfort, dizziness, or breathlessness. Perform the test on another day.

AEROBIC EFFICIENCY

STEP TEST

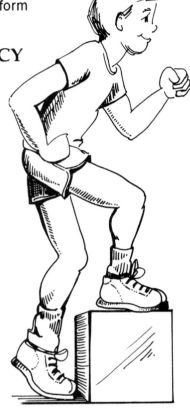

1. Select a bench, stool, or chair that is 12 inches high.
2. You will step up and down in an up, up, down, down brisk cadence.
3. Find a song that has a moderate tempo of about 96 beats per minute (16 beats in 10 seconds) to guide your cadence.
4. Rehearse the stepping with the music to get familiar with the pattern.
5. Practice finding your pulse on your wrist (on the inner edge of the wrist below the base of the thumb) or at your neck (below the ear along the jaw).
6. Now, perform the stepping for three continuous minutes. Upon completion of the time, immediately count your pulse for 10 seconds.

RESULTS OF THE STEP TEST
(Counting pulse for 10 seconds)

LEVEL	WOMEN	MEN	
EXCELLENT	16 or less	17 or less	Congratulations
GOOD	17–18	18–20	Keep it up!
FAIR	19–22	21–23	Begin or progress in an aerobic program.
POOR	23 or more	24 or more	Start with a moderate to easy aerobic program.

(Test based on the Harvard Step Test)

1.5 MILE RUN

1. Establish a distance of 1.5 miles. This is six laps around most school tracks (which are usually 1/4 mile).
2. Use a stopwatch to time yourself.
3. Warm up with some easy jogging and gentle stretching before you start.
4. Cover the distance as fast as you can (running/walking). Cool down gradually at the conclusion with brisk walking for several minutes.

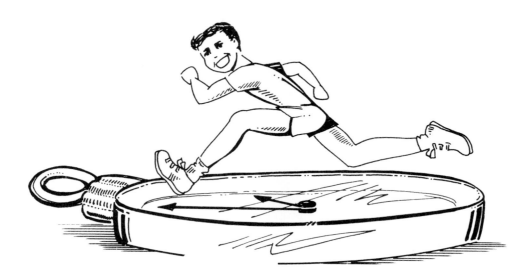

RESULTS OF THE 1.5 MILE RUN
Time (Minutes)

Fitness Category		13–19	20–29	Age (years) 30–39	40–49	50–59	60+
I. Very poor	(men)	> 15:31*	> 16:01	> 16:31	> 17:31	> 19:01	> 20:01
	(women)	> 18:31	> 19:01	> 19:31	> 20:01	> 20:31	> 21:01
II. Poor	(men)	12:11–15:30	14:01–16:00	14:44–16:30	15:36–17:30	17:01–19:00	19:01–20:00
	(women)	16:55–18:30	18:31–19:00	19:01–19:30	19:31–20:00	20:01–20:30	21:00–21:31
III. Fair	(men)	10:49–12:10	12:01–14:00	12:31–14:45	13:01–15:35	14:31–17:00	16:16–19:00
	(women)	14:31–16:54	15:55–18:30	16:31–19:00	17:31–19:30	19:01–20:00	19:31–20:30
IV. Good	(men)	9:41–10:48	10:46–12:00	11:01–12:30	11:31–13:00	12:31–14:30	14:00–16:15
	(women)	12:30–14:30	13:31–15:54	14:31–16:30	15:56–17:30	16:31–19:00	17:31–19:30
V. Excellent	(men)	8:37–9:40	9:45–10:45	10:00–11:00	10:30–11:30	11:00–12:30	11:15–13:59
	(women)	11:50–12:29	12:30–13:30	13:00–14:30	13:45–15:55	14:30–16:30	16:30–17:30
VI. Superior	(men)	< 8:37	< 9:45	< 10:00	< 10:30	< 11:00	< 11:15
	(women)	< 11:50	< 12:30	< 13:00	< 13:45	< 14:30	< 16:30

< Means "less than"; > means "more than."

From THE AEROBIC PROGRAM FOR TOTAL WELL-BEING by Kenneth H. Cooper. Copyright © 1982 by Kenneth H. Cooper. Reprinted by permission of Bantam Books, a division of Bantam, Doubleday, Dell, Publishing Group Inc.

ROCKPORT FITNESS WALKING TEST

The Rockport Walking Institute has developed a walking test to assess cardiorespiratory fitness for men and women ages 20–69. You are instructed to walk 1.0 mile as quickly and as comfortably as possible, and to take a heart rate immediately at the end of the test by counting the pulse for 15 seconds and multiplying that number by four (to get the heart rate for one minute). It is important that you take an accurate pulse. Make sure the course you walk on is flat, uninterrupted, and correctly measured. A quarter-mile track would be preferable.

You can use the Rockport relative fitness charts to classify your cardiorespiratory fitness. The walking time and corresponding post-exercise heart rate are located on the appropriate chart for your age and gender. These charts are based on body weights of 125 lb. for women and 170 lb. for men. If you weigh substantially more than this value, your cardiorespiratory fitness level will be overestimated.

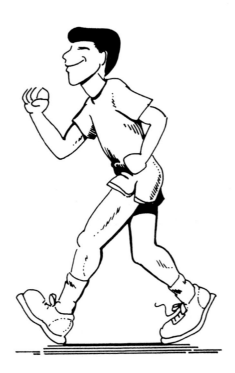

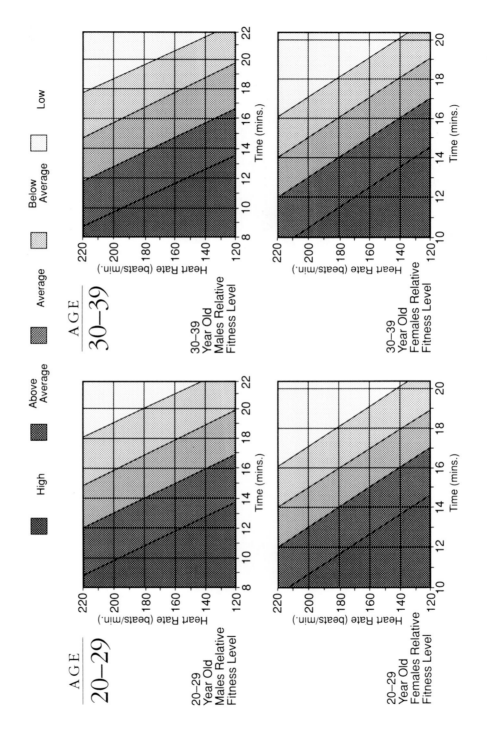

AGE
20–29

AGE
30–39

High

Above Average

Average

Below Average

Low

20–29 Year Old Males Relative Fitness Level

20–29 Year Old Females Relative Fitness Level

30–39 Year Old Males Relative Fitness Level

30–39 Year Old Females Relative Fitness Level

Heart Rate (beats/min.)

Time (mins.)

11

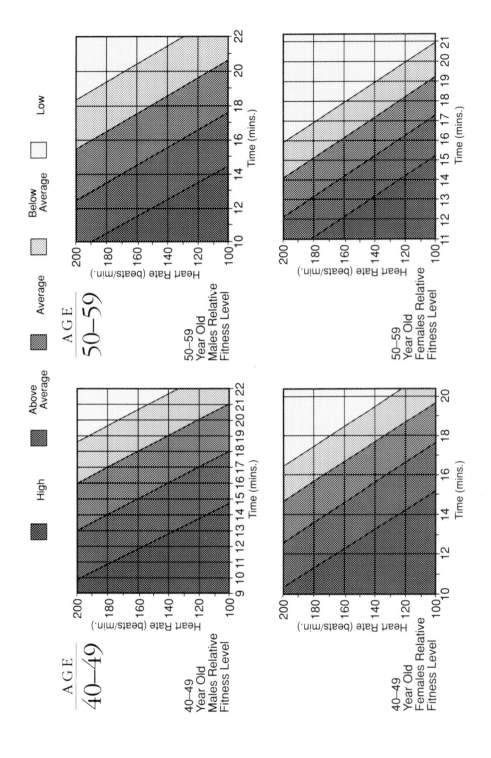

AGE
40–49

High   Above Average   Average   Below Average   Low

AGE
50–59

40–49 Year Old Males Relative Fitness Level

40–49 Year Old Females Relative Fitness Level

50–59 Year Old Males Relative Fitness Level

50–59 Year Old Females Relative Fitness Level

Heart Rate (beats/min.)

Time (mins.)

12

MUSCULAR STRENGTH AND ENDURANCE

ABDOMINAL STRENGTH AND ENDURANCE TEST

1. Lie on your back with your hands either supporting your head or across your chest.
2. Keep your legs bent at the knees, with the feet flat on the floor about six to ten inches from your buttocks.
3. To perform the "crunch," curl your trunk so that your shoulder blades come off the floor. (Your lower back stays on the floor.) Keep it smooth.
4. To take the test, count the number of "crunches" you can do for one minute.

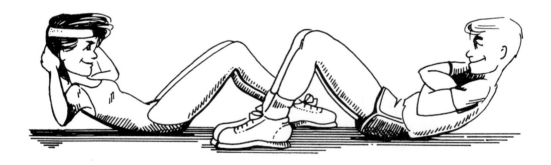

RESULTS FOR WOMEN AND MEN

CATEGORY	RESULTS
EXCELLENT	60 crunches or more
VERY GOOD	50 to 59 crunches
GOOD	42 to 49 crunches
FAIR	34 to 41 crunches
POOR	Less than 34 crunches

UPPER TORSO STRENGTH AND ENDURANCE TEST

The push-up may be completed in the standard style (with the body straight and supported by the hands and feet) or the modified style (with the knees on the ground).

1. Lower the chest so it almost makes contact with the floor and then straighten the arms.
2. To take the test, count the total number of push-ups completed in one minute.
3. Start with the modified push-up. Once you have reached the "excellent level" with the modified push-up, proceed to the standard push-up.

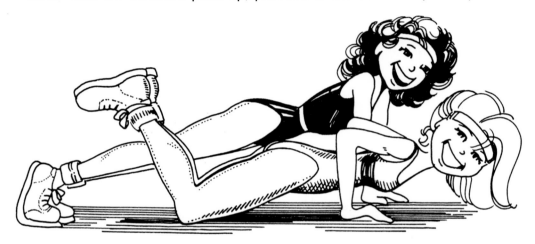

RESULTS

MODIFIED PUSH-UPS FOR WOMEN AND MEN	
EXCELLENT (GO TO STANDARD PUSH-UP)	32 push-ups or more
VERY GOOD	25 to 31 push-ups
GOOD	14 to 24 push-ups
FAIR	8 to 13 push-ups
POOR	Less than 8 push-ups

STANDARD PUSH-UPS FOR WOMEN AND MEN	
EXCELLENT	49 push-ups or more
VERY GOOD	39 to 48 push-ups
GOOD	28 to 38 push-ups
FAIR	15 to 27 push-ups
POOR	Less than 15 push-ups

FLEXIBILITY

SIT AND REACH TEST

Flexibility is specific. This means that the degree of flexibility in one joint will not necessarily be the same in other joints of the body. Since a lack of flexibility in the lower back, back of the legs, and hips is a contributing cause for 80% of lower back problems of our population, this flexibility test was chosen.

1. Sit with your legs extended in front of you. Keep your feet perpendicular to the floor. Place a ruler along your legs on the floor.
2. Slowly stretch forward, reaching towards (or past) your toes and hold. (Do not bounce!) Keep your legs straight but not locked.
3. It is best to do this several times for practice, gently stretching further towards your point of limitation.

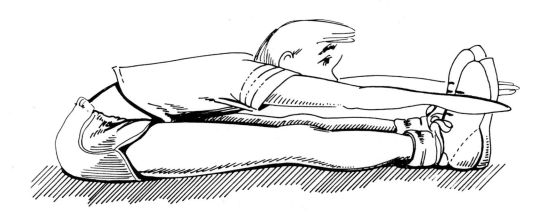

RESULTS OF THE SIT AND REACH TEST FOR WOMEN AND MEN

CATEGORY	RESULTS
EXCELLENT	7 inches or more past the toes
VERY GOOD	4 to 7 inches past the toes
GOOD	1 to 4 inches past the toes
FAIR	2 inches from in front of the toes to 1 inch past
POOR	More than 2 inches in front of the toes

This sit and reach test does not differentiate between a person with short arms and/or long legs and someone with long arms and/or short legs. Therefore the test results should be interpreted accordingly.

BODY COMPOSITION

PINCH TEST FOR BODY FAT

The pinch test is a quick check for body composition. (You can always count on the mirror to tell you a lot, too!)

1. With your thumb and forefinger, pinch the skin and fat at the waist just above the hips. (Be sure not to pinch any muscle. Pull the skinfold away from your body.)
2. With a ruler measure the width of the pinch.

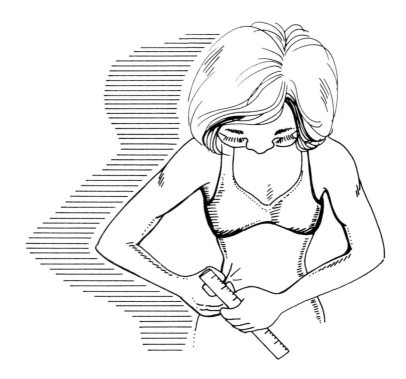

RESULTS OF PINCH TEST

LEVEL	MEN	WOMEN
GOOD TO EXCELLENT	1/2 inch or less	1 inch or less
FAIR TO GOOD	1 inch to 1/2	1 1/2 inch to 1 inch
POOR	Over 1 inch	Over 1 1/2 inch

Refer to SKINFOLD CALIPER MEASUREMENT for a more accurate estimate of body composition.

BODY COMPOSITION
SKINFOLD CALIPER MEASUREMENT

Approximately one-half of the fat in the body is located just under the skin and is closely correlated to total body fat. Researchers have demonstrated that this skinfold fat is distributed differently in men and women and, for that reason, skinfold measurements are taken at different body locations. Skinfolds should not be taken immediately after exercise, because the shift of body fluids will increase the skinfold size.

There are several practical and inexpensive skinfold calipers available for body composition analysis. To take a skinfold measurement, grasp the anatomical site with the thumb and index finger. Lift the skinfold away from the site to make sure no muscle is caught in the fold. Place the caliper one-half to one inch below the thumb and index finger. Allow the caliper to stabilize for a few seconds before reading. Take at least three measurements and record the average. Total the average of your skinfolds. Determine your percentage of body fat by placing a straight edge from your age to the sum of the three skinfolds on the nomogram. The recommended percentage of body fat is 16 to 25 percent for a woman and 12 to 18 percent for a man. There is an error factor of plus or minus three to five percent with skinfold body composition assessment.

Skinfolds are conventionally taken on the right side of the body. Here is how to find the anatomical skinfold sites:

Chest—the fold over the side border of the pectoralis major

Abdomen—vertical fold adjacent to the umbilicus

Thigh—vertical fold on the front part of the thigh midway between the hip and knee joint

Triceps—vertical fold on the back of the arm midway between the shoulder and elbow (arm held straight and relaxed)

Suprailium—diagonal fold above the crest of the ilium

ANATOMICAL SKINFOLD SITES

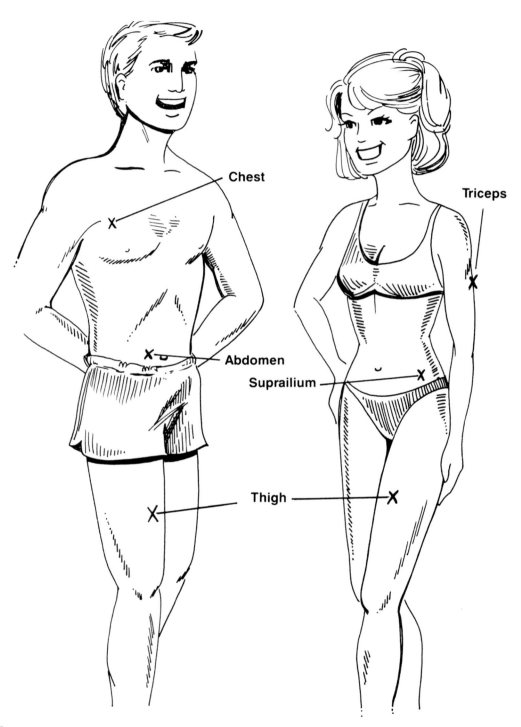

Chest

Triceps

Abdomen

Suprailium

Thigh

SKINFOLD NOMOGRAM

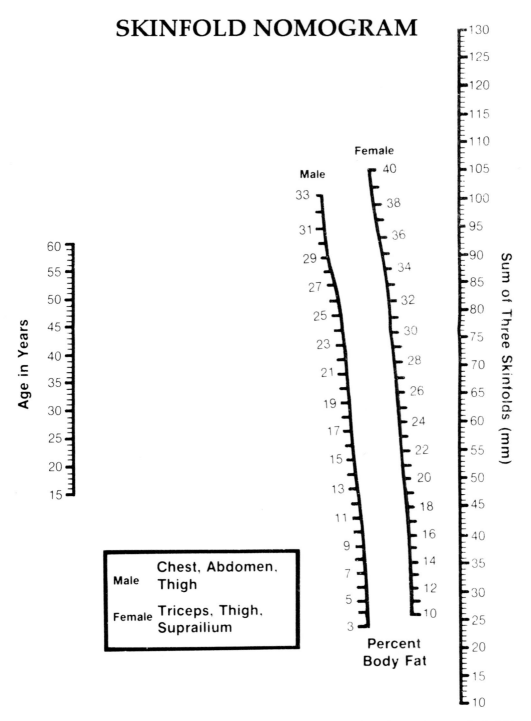

Reprinted by permission from Baun, W.B. and Baun, M.R. A nomogram for the estimate of percent body fat from generalized equations. *Research Quarterly for Exercise and Sport,* 1981, 52, 380–384.

THE "S.P.O.R.T." PRINCIPLE

Fitness conditioning involves the "S.P.O.R.T." principle: Specificity, Progression, Overload, Reversibility, and Training Effect.

SPECIFICITY: Specificity takes the guesswork out of training. Your body will adapt to the specific type of training you choose. If you want to run marathons, you've got to train long distances. If you wish to build muscles, you must do intense weight training. Identify your goals and get started.

PROGRESSION: Challenge your body's abilities gradually. Let your body adapt to its new capability and then you can progress some more. (Injuries happen from trying to do too much, too soon, too hard, and too fast.)

OVERLOAD: You "overload" by increasing the intensity, duration, or frequency of your established level of exercise. For instance, you may do aerobics longer, more times a week, or at a more intense level. When your exercise program becomes easier and somewhat routine it is often a good time to overload. Overload your exercise program in increments of 10 percent of your present ability.

REVERSIBILITY: You can't **store** exercise. If you stop exercising there is a marked decrease in skill, endurance, strength, etc. from your previous level. So keep it up!

TRAINING EFFECT: As you specifically train for a certain activity, you gradually and progressively overload your body's ability. The resulting increase in muscular and cardiorespiratory conditioning is the training effect.

Your final phase is to **MAINTAIN** this newly acquired level of health throughout your lifetime. You can do it!

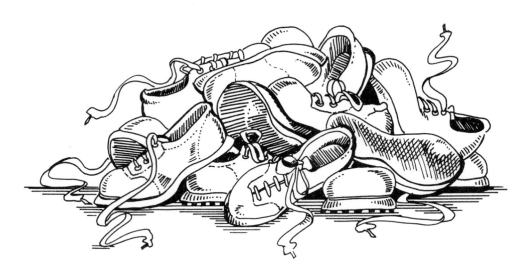

THE FORMULA FOR AEROBIC FITNESS

Recent statistics indicate that only one-third of all adults exercise regularly enough to promote optimal fitness. To benefit from a sound cardiorespiratory program follow the "F.I.T." formula. "F.I.T." stands for Frequency, Intensity, and Time.

FREQUENCY: For optimal results, perform your aerobic activity three to five times a week (preferably every other day). If you choose to exercise more, make sure you rest at least one day each week to prevent any injuries from overuse!

INTENSITY: Your intensity should be 60 percent to 85 percent of your personalized training zone. For beginners in good health, 60 percent to 70 percent of your training zone is encouraged.

TIME: The time or duration should gradually build up to between 20 and 60 minutes.

HEART RATE MONITORING

Monitoring your heart rate is a very simple, practical, and safe way to understand your exertion during aerobics. You will improve your cardiorespiratory system if you train at 60 percent to 85 percent of your personalized target zone. To estimate your target zone, you must first calculate your maximum heart rate and your resting heart rate. Your maximum heart rate (the fastest your heart will beat) can be estimated by subtracting your age from 220. Resting heart rate is defined as the average heart rate (per minute) prior to initiating any physical activity. It is often measured in the morning, after waking up and prior to physical activity. Here's how a 30-year-old individual with a resting heart rate of 72 would estimate her personalized target zone.

Constant:	220	
Your age:	−30	
Subtract age from constant; this equals estimated maximum heart rate:	= 190	
Your resting heart rate:	−72	
Subtract resting heart rate from estimated maximum heart rate:	= 118	
Multiply by:	60%	85%
Equals:	71	100
Add resting heart rate from	+72	+72
Equals exercise heart rate:	143	172
	TARGET ZONE	

PERSONALIZED TARGET ZONE

Constant:	220	
Your age:		
Subtract age from constant; this equals estimated maximum heart rate:		
Your resting heart rate:		
Subtract resting heart rate from estimated maximum heart rate:		
Multiply by:	60%	85%
Equals:		
Add resting heart rate:		
Equals exercise heart rate:		
	TARGET ZONE	

Find your pulse on your wrist (on the inner edge of the wrist below the base of the thumb) or neck (below the ear along the jaw) and count for 10 seconds and then multiply by six to find the beats per minute. Pulse monitoring at the wrist is recommended because you can inadvertently press too hard on the neck and cause a slowing of the heart rate (with some people)! Monitor your heart rate before, after three to five minutes of aerobic exercise, and upon completion of an aerobic section.

You can also monitor exercise intensity through the use of perceived exertion. With perceived exertion you interpret various body sensations such as heart rate, muscle and joint sensations, breathing intensity, and body temperature, and subjectively estimate your exercise intensity. A model that corresponds exercise heart rate with perceived exertion has been developed by Gunnar Borg, a Swedish physiologist. Notice that by adding a "0" to the numbers of the perceived exertion scale it correlates to your exercise heart rate intensity. This is a great way to learn to listen to your body and compare your results to your counted heart rate. An easy way to know if you are within your ideal aerobic exercise intensity is to perceptually monitor your breathing intensity. If you are aware of a deeper and more frequent breathing pattern but are not hyperventilating and can still talk to an exercise partner, you are probably exercising within the desired aerobic exercise intensity range.

RATE OF PERCEIVED EXERTION SCALE		
6	14	
7 Very, very light	15	Hard
8	16	
9 Very light	17	Very hard
10	18	
11 Fairly light	19	Very, very hard
12	20	
13 Somewhat hard		

From Borg, G. "Perceived Exertion: A Note on History and Methods." *Medicine and Science in Sports and Exercise* 5:90–93, 1983.

FINDING YOUR PULSE

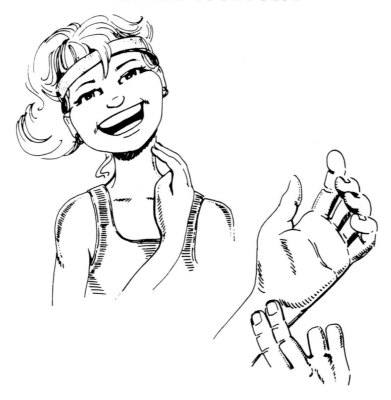

THE TEN COMMANDMENTS
OF BODY SHAPING

Doing your exercises is not enough. It's doing them right that really counts. Follow these 10 commandments for effective results.

1. **CONTROL YOUR MOVEMENT.** Avoid fast, jerky movements which rely too heavily on momentum and may be harmful to your muscles and joints.
2. **PERFORM ALL EXERCISES THROUGH THE COMPLETE RANGE OF MOTION.** The benefits of strength, endurance, flexibility, skill, and performance are best achieved when exercises are performed through the full range of movement. Sometimes small range-of-motion movements are incorporated with the full range movements. (Exception: to avoid stressing the neck, do not take the head straight back.)
3. **ALWAYS EXERCISE OPPOSING MUSCLE GROUPS.** You need to balance the strength of opposing muscles. (See THE MUSCLE SYSTEM for a list of opposing muscle groups.)
4. **CONCENTRATE ON THE MUSCLES YOU ARE WORKING.** Focusing on the specific muscle groups you are working will help you to know when and how much to overload.
5. **DO THE EXERCISES PROPERLY.** The quality, form, and technique of the exercise is very important. Don't just try to see how many repetitions of an exercise you can do!
6. **BREATHE NORMALLY.** Always **exhale** as you **exert.** Do not hold your breath!
7. **DON'T EXERCISE TO THE POINT OF PAIN.** Pain is a warning sign—STOP before you hurt yourself.
8. **VARY YOUR PROGRAM AND EXERCISES.** This prevents boredom, staleness, and overtraining.
9. **EXERCISE MAJOR BODY PARTS EARLY IN THE WORKOUT.** Work your larger muscle groups, such as your legs and chest, before isolating your smaller muscle groups. That way the fatigue in the smaller muscle groups will not affect the performance of the heavier, more difficult exercises.
10. **BE FAITHFUL TO YOUR WARM-UP AND COOL-DOWN ROUTINES.** You **need** them to prevent injuries and reduce muscle soreness. And keep moving during the workout to keep your muscles pliable.

TRAINING TIPS

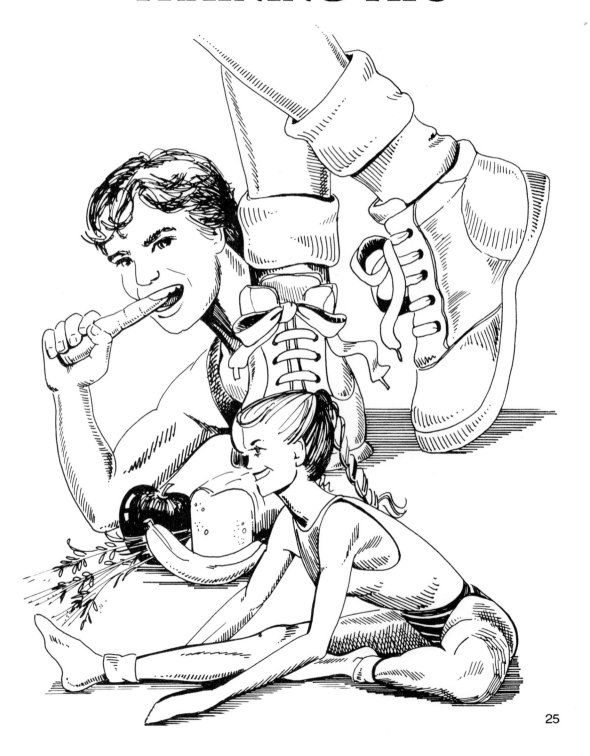

MAXIMIZE YOUR RESULTS, MINIMIZE YOUR RISKS

Not all exercises are good for you. Here are some unsafe or poorly executed exercises with their preferred alternatives.

1) **TWISTING HOPS**
   The combination of twisting the spine while hopping on the floor can be quite stressful on the back. The force of hopping alone equals two to three times your body weight.

   ALTERNATIVE: Jump rope hops do not require any twisting and are more controllable.

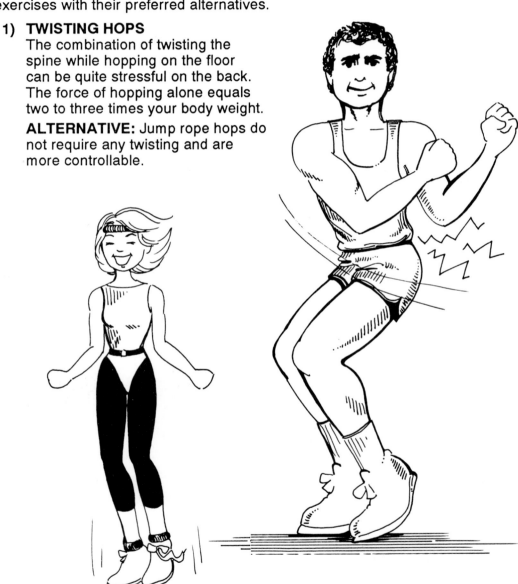

2) FAST-TWISTING WAIST EXERCISES

The fast side-to-side twisting of the torso imposes a shearing stress on the vertebrae of the spine.

ALTERNATIVE: Do them **slowly** as a warm-up stretch. Twisting crunches are more effective waist work.

3) TOE TOUCHES

This straight-legged position puts too much stretch on the ligaments behind the knees and stresses the lower spine. Bouncing touches are even worse!

ALTERNATIVE: The seated pike stretch (with slightly bent knees) and the seated half-straddle stretch are much better for you.

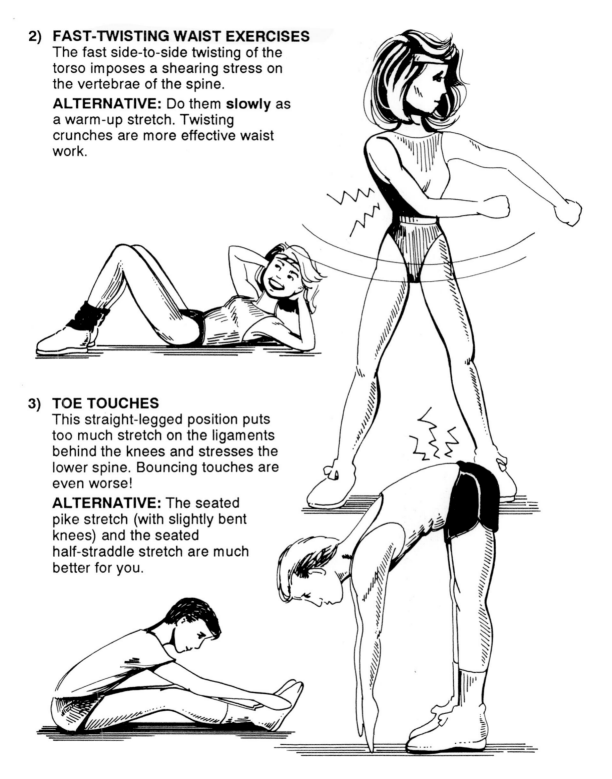

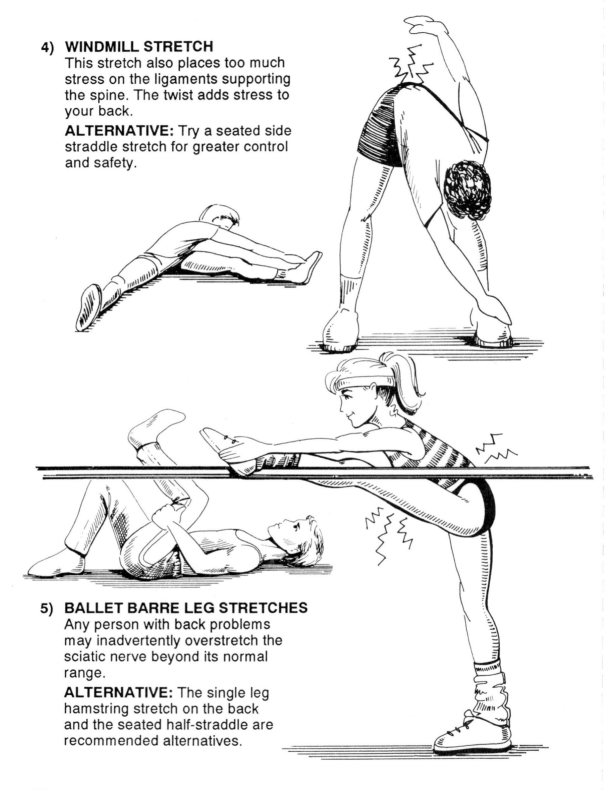

4) WINDMILL STRETCH

This stretch also places too much stress on the ligaments supporting the spine. The twist adds stress to your back.

ALTERNATIVE: Try a seated side straddle stretch for greater control and safety.

5) BALLET BARRE LEG STRETCHES

Any person with back problems may inadvertently overstretch the sciatic nerve beyond its normal range.

ALTERNATIVE: The single leg hamstring stretch on the back and the seated half-straddle are recommended alternatives.

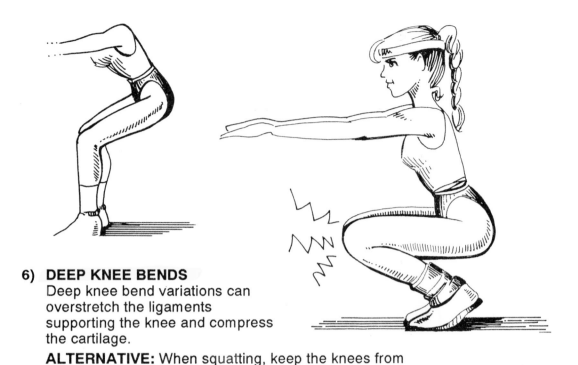

6) DEEP KNEE BENDS

Deep knee bend variations can overstretch the ligaments supporting the knee and compress the cartilage.

ALTERNATIVE: When squatting, keep the knees from protruding past the toes and lower your buttocks to just above your knees.

7) LUNGES WITH PROTRUDING KNEES

The lunge is often incorrectly performed. A bent knee which juts past the ankle places stress on the knee.

ALTERNATIVE: Make sure the front knee stays over the toes.

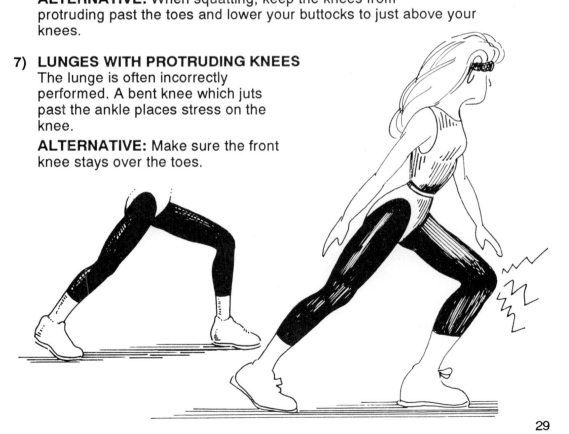

8) HURDLER'S STRETCH

This exercise can overstretch the muscles in the groin and the ligaments of the bent knee.

ALTERNATIVE: The seated center straddle stretch and half-straddle stretch are better options.

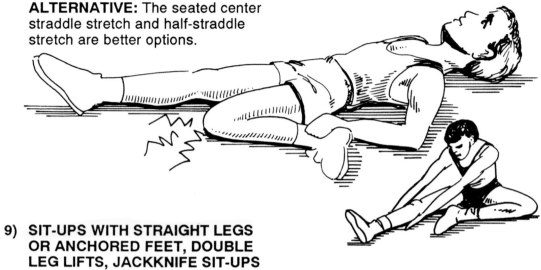

9) SIT-UPS WITH STRAIGHT LEGS OR ANCHORED FEET, DOUBLE LEG LIFTS, JACKKNIFE SIT-UPS

These exercises predominantly use the hip flexors (the muscles in front of the thigh which attach to the lower back), not the abdominals! Their repeated performance may lead to back problems.

ALTERNATIVE: Use the "crunch" variations which bring your ribs towards your pelvis as you lift only your shoulders and upper back off the floor.

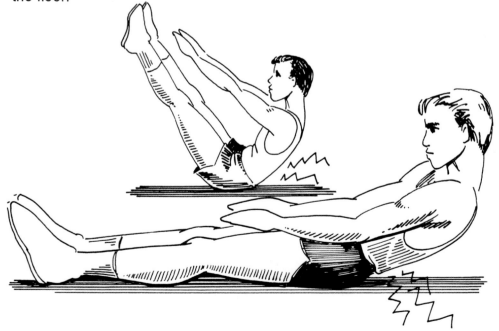

10) HEAD THROWS IN A CRUNCH
Often the head is "thrown forward" during a crunch.

ALTERNATIVE: Keep your head in a neutral position. Focus on the ceiling.

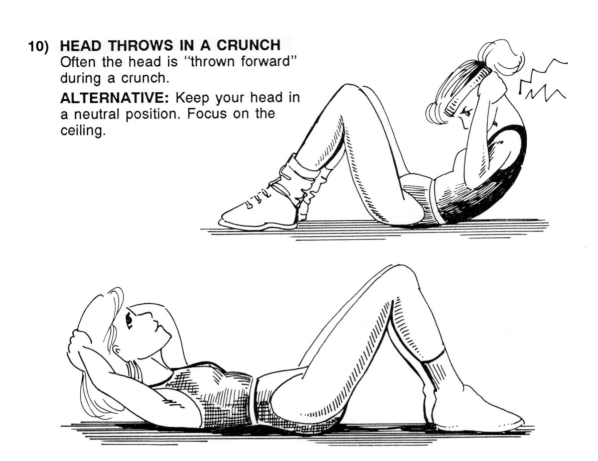

11) SWAN LIFTS
The combination of arching the lower spine as the muscles are contracting can injure the back.

ALTERNATIVE: Keep the lower body on the floor and only lift the upper body, as in the back extension. Or, lift one arm in front and the opposite leg in back. Repeat the movement lifting the opposite limbs.

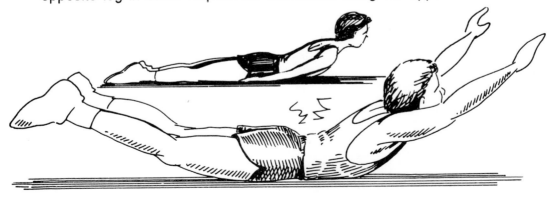

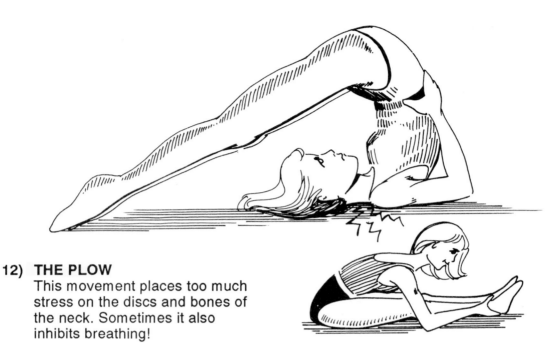

12) THE PLOW
This movement places too much stress on the discs and bones of the neck. Sometimes it also inhibits breathing!

ALTERNATIVE: The seated pike stretch (with soft knees) is more effective.

13) GYMNASTICS BRIDGES AND PELVIC LIFTS
The gymnastics bridge, designed to stretch the upper back and shoulders, is usually performed with an over-arched lower back. Pelvic lifts are frequently over-arched as well.

ALTERNATIVE: Use the prone prop or prone extension instead of the bridge. And be careful not to over-arch when performing the pelvic lift.

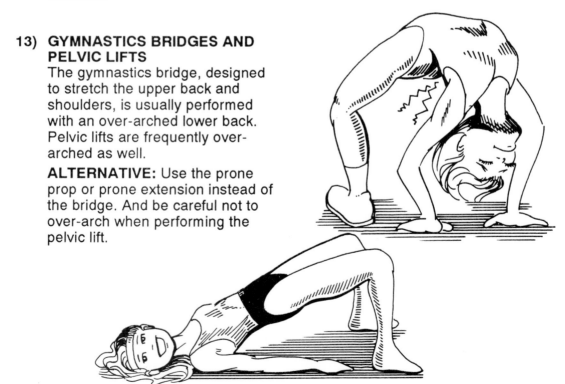

14) LEG LIFTING EXERCISES

Leg lifts or side leg exercises can twist and strain the lower back if they are done too fast.

ALTERNATIVE: Place your elbows on the floor, keep your back straight, and control the movement. Do not swing or fling legs.

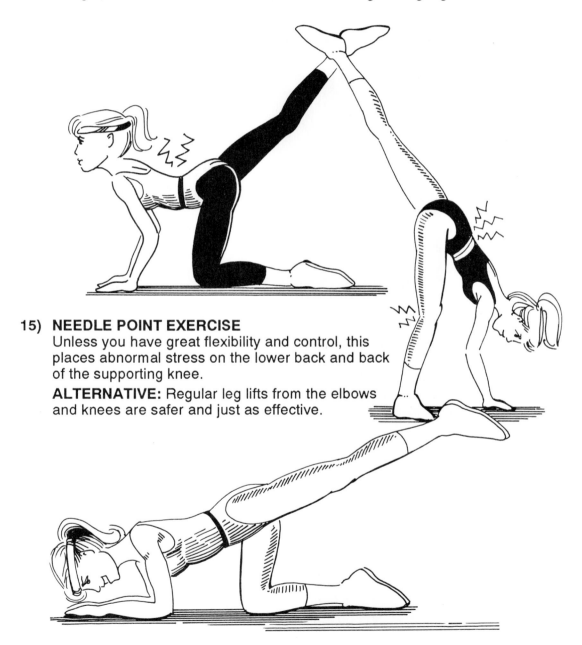

15) NEEDLE POINT EXERCISE

Unless you have great flexibility and control, this places abnormal stress on the lower back and back of the supporting knee.

ALTERNATIVE: Regular leg lifts from the elbows and knees are safer and just as effective.

33

16) SIDE STRADDLE STRETCH

If you allow the opposite hip to come off the floor while stretching to the side, you place the hip and spine in poor alignment.

ALTERNATIVE: Keep the buttocks and legs firmly on the floor.

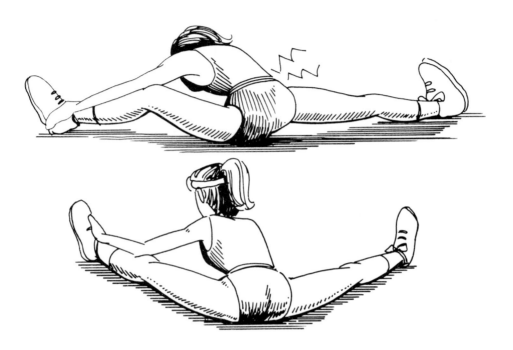

THE MOST COMMON MISTAKES IN EXERCISE

The following are some of the most common mistakes that occur in exercise programs.

1) OVERTRAINING: In their zeal to achieve fitness, people often try too hard. Possible signs of overtraining are: injury, weight loss, mental dullness, disturbed digestion, loss of appetite, early exhaustion during a workout, fatigue during the day, or elevated heart rate upon rising or after a workout. Stress quality, not quantity!

2) POOR EXERCISE TECHNIQUE: Exercises performed incorrectly can lead to injury and poor performance. Poor technique is most frequent during the latter stages of a workout.

3) IMPROPER EQUIPMENT: The exercise clothes you wear, the shoes on your feet, the surface you are training on, and the equipment you are using can all **improve** or **impair** your performance.

4) INSUFFICIENT WARM-UP: Too often, the main activity is begun without proper warm-up (or after a quick, insufficient warm-up). This can lead to injury.

5) **EXTRA-LONG WORKOUTS:** See signs of overtraining.

6) **LIFTING WEIGHTS THAT ARE TOO HEAVY:** This leads to improper exercise technique, predisposes you to injury, and is not the progressive overload needed for optimal results in strength and endurance. Realize your limits.

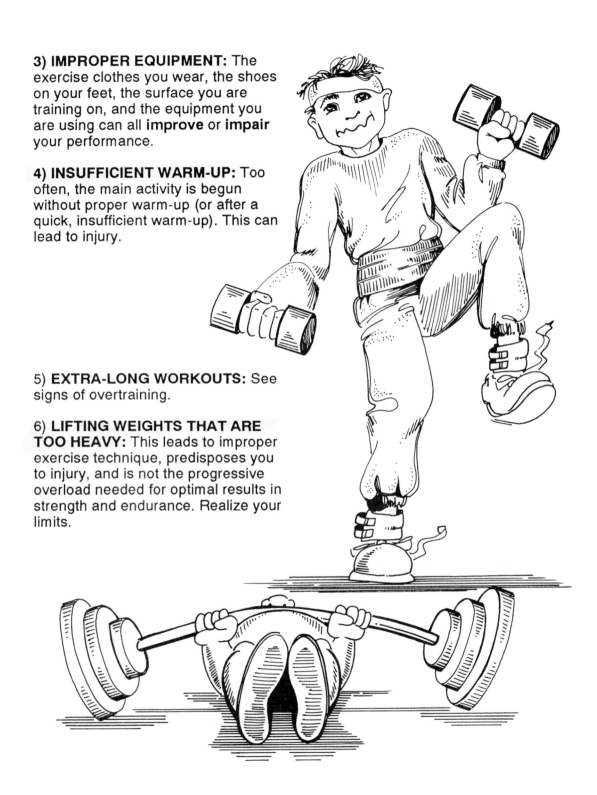

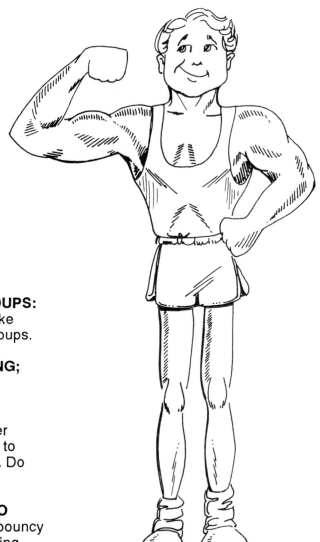

7) FORGETTING MUSCLE GROUPS:
For complete body symmetry make
sure you work **all** your muscle groups.

8) UNREALISTIC GOAL-SETTING;
Set realistic short- and long-term
goals.

9) FORCED BREATHING: Proper
breathing during exercise is easy to
remember—**exhale** as you **exert.** Do
not force your breathing.

**10) EXERCISES THAT ARE TOO
BOUNCY AND FAST:** Fast and bouncy
movements stimulate your opposing
muscle groups to contract and hinder
the movement. Control is the key!

11) INADEQUATE AEROBIC COOL-DOWN: Blood pressure may drop
significantly from an abrupt cessation of vigorous aerobic exercise. This
may also lead to fainting and irregular heart beats. Slow down gradually;
don't just stop!

12) INSUFFICIENT STRETCHING AT THE END OF THE WORKOUT: Slow
stretching following a workout helps reduce muscle soreness and improve
flexibility.

IN CASE OF INJURY

Let's face it. When you pursue an active lifestyle, you will occasionally overdo it. And even if you are careful, inadequate equipment (such as poor aerobic shoes) or exercising on an improper surface can lead to injuries. You can usually tell when you have an injury; pain and swelling appear in an area and gradually worsen. What do you do? R.I.C.E. (Rest, Ice, Compression, Elevation) is the answer. Most of these problems are muscle, ligament, and tendon injuries. The R.I.C.E. approach will limit the injury and accelerate the healing.

Rest prevents you from re-injury and decreases the circulation to the area. "Time heals."

Ice should be applied immediately to the injured area to keep the swelling down. An ice pack may be applied for 10 to 20 minutes periodically through the first 24 hours. Direct ice massage can be used for 7 to 10 minute sessions with the same effects. Heat can be applied after 48 hours, in conjunction with ice, to increase the circulation and enhance the body's process of removing the excess blood and fluid.

Compression helps reduce the swelling and internal bleeding. Ace bandages are a good way to do this. Be careful not to obstruct circulation by over-tightening!

Elevation helps reduce the internal bleeding and excessive fluid entry to the injury. If possible, elevate the injured area above the level of the heart at all opportune times until the swelling subsides.

See your physician if necessary. Persistent pain, major swelling, and significant discoloration all require elevation. The **cause** of the injury must also be **corrected** so re-injury does not occur. (Maybe you need new shoes, less weight, shorter workouts, etc.) Begin your rehabilitation process of stretching and strengthening and return to your former level of activity when your body is READY!

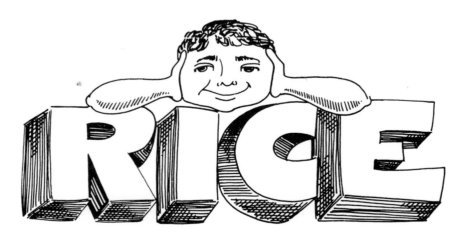

COMMON AEROBIC INJURIES

The most common aerobic injury is a pain between the knee and ankle, commonly referred to as "shin splints." Shin pain can be caused by a number of conditions, but impact shock is probably the major cause. Rest, ice, and exercise to increase muscle strength/flexibility are standard treatments. Footwear (specifically the arch support), floor surface resiliency, movement selection, and the structure of the workout should be reevaluated for safety and effectiveness. If this pain continues, see your physician.

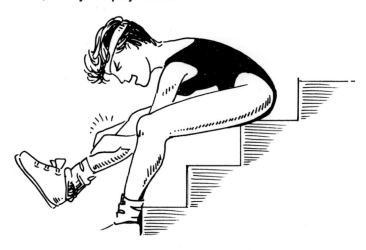

A variety of knee injuries which affect the joint structure may also occur in aerobic exercise. Repeated floor impact and rolling on the foot inward upon impact can contribute to these problems. Proper footwear, resilient workout surface, sufficient warm-up, and the progressive increase in exercise intensity will help to prevent these injuries.

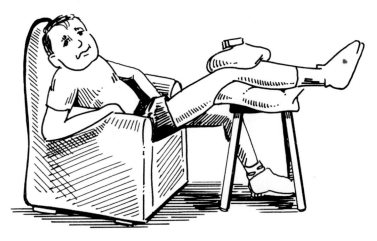

An ankle sprain is another common injury. It usually occurs when the weak ligaments on the outside of the joint are injured by an accidental rolling outward of the ankle. Rest, ice, compression, and elevation are standard treatments; physician referral may be necessary. Safe movement selection, proper warm-up, and concentration on the activity itself will help prevent this type of injury.

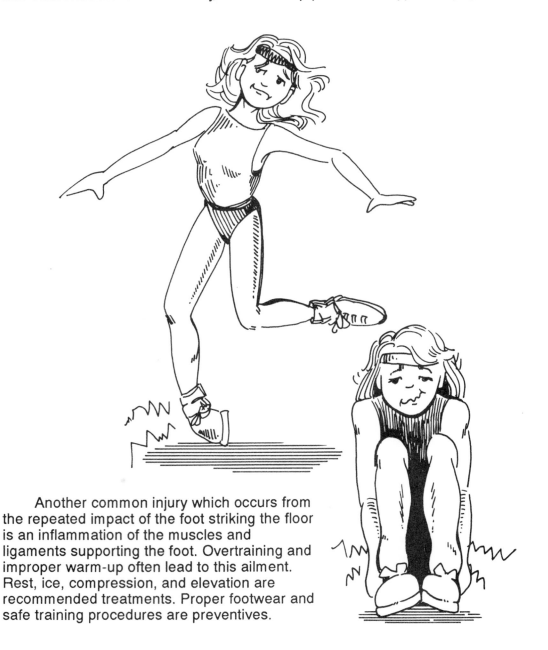

Another common injury which occurs from the repeated impact of the foot striking the floor is an inflammation of the muscles and ligaments supporting the foot. Overtraining and improper warm-up often lead to this ailment. Rest, ice, compression, and elevation are recommended treatments. Proper footwear and safe training procedures are preventives.

GUIDE TO A BETTER BACK

It's a pain! But almost everyone encounters a lower back problem sometime. What can you do to prevent back problems? Use your back correctly for daily activities, improve your posture, stretch and strengthen your abdominal muscles, and control your weight.

THE DO'S TO FOLLOW

STANDING AND WALKING

Maintain your normal back curve, but avoid the swayback posture. Stand tall, feeling lifted throughout the lower abdominal region. Try not to stand still too long. If you must, put one leg up on a support or at least bend alternate knees. Limit your high heel wearing time since these shoes accentuate the back curve and create stress on the spine. Use your abdominal muscles to support your body weight as you stand or move.

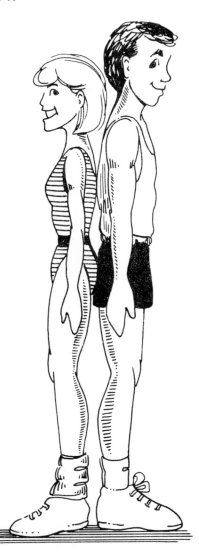

LIFTING

Bend your knees, not your back, when lifting. Hold objects close to your body and avoid over-the-head lifts. Avoid rotating your body when lifting or lowering an object. Instead, change your foot placement while maintaining the object directly in front of you.

SITTING AND DRIVING

Sit in firm-backed chairs with your feet flat on the floor. A small towel roll may be used behind the lower back to maintain an erect sitting posture. Placing your feet on a stool is fine, just avoid slumping or over-arching your back. In your car, move the seat forward so you don't have to stretch for the pedals and round your back. Men, bulging wallets in your hip pocket can lead to back and leg discomfort!

SLEEPING

Try sleeping on your side on a firm mattress with your knees slightly bent or on your back with a pillow under your knees. If you must sleep on your stomach, place a small pillow under your abdominals to correct for a sagging spine.

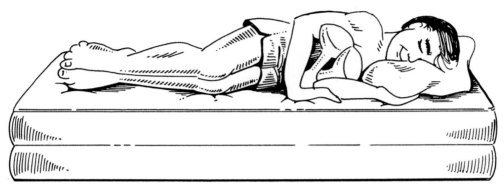

TEST YOUR POSTURE

With correct posture you maintain the normal curve in the lower back. Test your posture by standing with your hips, back, and head against the wall. Your heels should be a couple of inches away. There should be only minimal space between your lower back and the wall. You should be standing tall with a long neck and eyes straight forward.

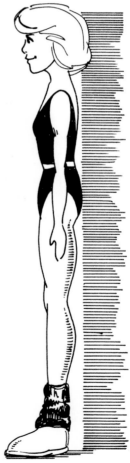

BACK PAIN RELIEF

Back injuries require the attention of a specialist. For relief of small arches, lie on your back on a padded surface and elevate your feet (with bent knees) on a padded chair. Place a small pillow or rolled-up towel under your neck and rest in this position for 10 to 15 minutes.

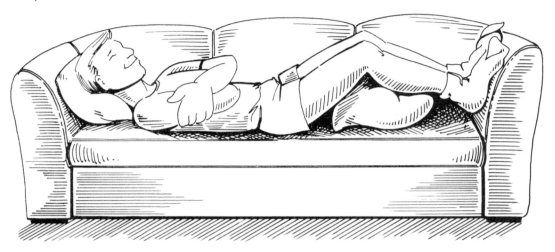

EXERCISES FOR A HEALTHY BACK

1. PELVIC TILT: Lie on your back with knees bent, arms on chest, and feet on floor. Press the lower back into the floor by tightening the abdominal muscles and slightly lifting the buttocks off the floor. Hold for 10 seconds and repeat 8 to 15 times.

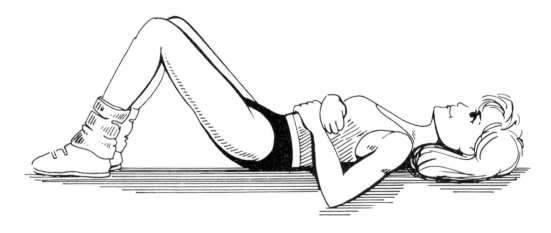

2. HAMSTRING/LOWER BACK STRETCH: Lie on your back, with both knees bent and one foot on the floor. Grasp behind the lifted knee, bring it towards the chest, and hold for several seconds. Repeat 3 to 5 times on each leg.

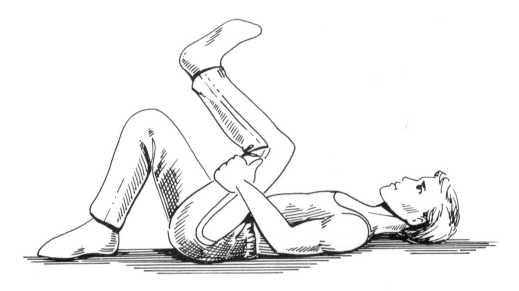

3. TUCK-HOLD: Tuck both knees to chest and slowly tighten tuck with arms while you press your lower back into floor. Keep your back flat. Hold for 10 seconds and repeat 5 to 10 times.

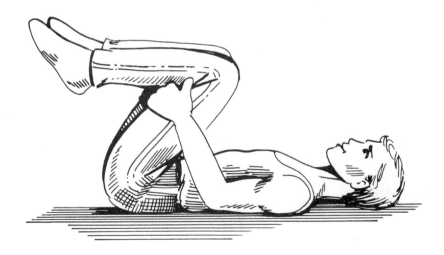

4. SLOW CRUNCH: Lie on your back with your knees bent at a 45 degree angle and your head supported at the base of the neck by your hands. Slowly lift your chest as you press your lower back into the floor; then slowly lower. Try lifting your buttocks slightly off the floor as you raise the chest. Repeat 8 to 25 times.

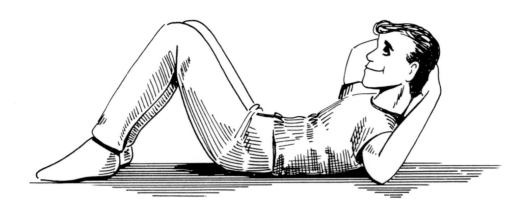

5. PRONE PROP: While on your stomach, lift your chest off the floor and hold by propping your elbows on the ground.

VARIATION: Same as prone prop, only straighten your arms. For both, relax your hips and abdominals and hold for several seconds and then lower. Repeat 3 to 5 times.

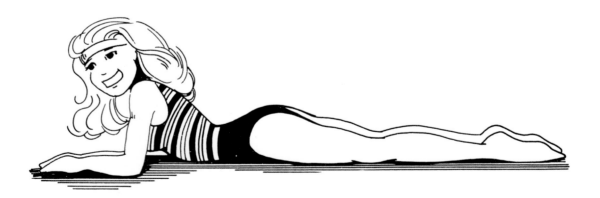

THE ALL-AROUND BEST-BALANCED EATING PLAN

Include a variety of wholesome foods in your total dietary intake. "Wholesome food" refers to food consumed in its natural state (or as close to its natural state as possible and free of additives, preservatives, or artificial ingredients) such as baked potatoes vs. potato chips; raw fruits and vegetables instead of cooked and canned varieties; and whole-grain breads and cereals as compared to refined products. Processing often removes important nutrients. The best way to obtain the most vitamins and minerals is to eat food in its natural form.

The all-around best-balanced diet contains adequate amounts of carbohydrates, protein, fats, vitamins, minerals, and water.

CARBOHYDRATES

Carbohydrates are the primary and most easily utilized source of energy for your body. Approximately 58 percent of your total caloric intake should come from carbohydrates. Refined and simple sugars, starches (complex carbohydrates), and fiber (cellulose) are the three forms in which carbohydrates are found in your food products. Refined sugars should be limited to approximately 10 percent of your daily carbohydrate intake. Complex carbohydrates, in the form of starches and naturally occurring simple sugars, should comprise the 48 percent balance of caloric intake from the carbohydrate food group. These are readily found in whole grain breads, vegetables, and fruit. Your body uses carbohydrates, in the form of glycogen and glucose, to provide the energy for moderate, prolonged, and intense exercise, and to contribute to the maintenance and functioning of your nervous system. In addition, under normal conditions, carbohydrates are the only energy source for your brain.

PROTEINS

Proteins are important for the healthy building and repair of every cell of your body. The essential amino acids, which cannot be manufactured within your body, must come from dietary sources. Twelve percent of your daily caloric intake should come from protein sources containing the essential amino acids. Americans tend to consume about twice as much protein as they actually need. Among key points to remember regarding protein are the following: 1) Proteins are important in helping to maintain your body's water balance. 2) Proteins in the blood help keep the acid level of the blood within a normal range. 3) Proteins are essential for you to have an immune response. This response produces antibodies to foreign substances that get into your system. 4) Many of your hormones are either protein or have protein components. 5) All of the many enzymes of your body are proteins. 6) Proteins act as carriers for a number of substances in your body. 7) Proteins play a role of passing information across spaces between nerves and muscles.

FATS

The biggest dietary challenge for most Americans is to reduce fat consumption. Total dietary calories from fat sources should be no more than 30 percent of daily food intake. Fats come in three important dietary forms: saturated, monounsaturated, and polyunsaturated. Saturated fats are found in animal products, including meats, poultry, and dairy products such as milk and cheeses. Tropical oils such as palm oil are predominantly saturated fat and are found in many prepared products. Saturated fat intake should be limited to less than 10 percent of daily caloric intake. The monounsaturated fats such as olive oil and polyunsaturated fats such as sunflower oil should comprise 10 percent each of daily caloric intake. You need some dietary fat and cholesterol to provide insulation, for energy, for the production of some hormones, for absorption of certain vitamins, and as a vital component of cell walls.

Unfortunately, elevated blood levels of fat have been linked to diseases of the cardiovascular system and to some forms of cancer. The typical American diet contains over 45 percent of calories from fat. The process of reducing this level is difficult and probably more likely to be successfully changed when done slowly. However, the results in potentially better health are well worth the effort invested.

WATER

Water is your most vital nutrient. Over 70 percent of lean body mass is water, while only 20 percent of body fat is water. Thus, lean body mass is mostly water and fat is mostly fat. Water is an important constituent of all body cells. It surrounds the cells, permeates bone tissue, and is the foundation element of the circulatory system. Among its important functions are transportation of nutrients, removal of the by-products of cell metabolism, temperature regulation, joint lubrication, and cell structure shape. In addition, water is a medium for life-sustaining chemical reactions in the body.

48

VITAMINS

A well-balanced diet does not have to be supplemented to meet the daily vitamin requirements. However, a deficiency of one or more vitamins will result in some kind of symptom or deficiency reaction, while too much of a vitamin may cause a toxic reaction. Vitamins are grouped into two groups based on their solubility. There are the water soluble vitamins (B vitamins and C) and the fat-soluble vitamins (A, D, E, K). Toxicity is more likely to occur with fat soluble than with water soluble vitamins. The best way to get vitamins in your body is from the foods you eat. Avoid low nutrient foods like soft drinks and foods high in calories and fat. Nutrient dense foods like whole grains and fresh fruits and vegetables will provide adequate daily caloric intake, as well as vitamins and other micronutrients. Beliefs that extra amounts of certain vitamins will give extra energy, reduce stress, prevent a variety of ailments, or improve endurance has not been proven by controlled research.

MINERALS

The minerals, or micronutrients, are inorganic substances which your body needs in small amounts each day. They facilitate numerous functions in your bodily processes such as enzymatic activities, electrolyte balance, and fluid transport. They also have structural roles in the body.

Following are some general eating guidelines to help you design your all-around best-balanced eating plan.

MEAT AND PROTEIN FOODS

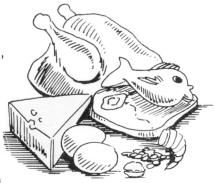

Eat less red meat; reduce the serving size and frequency.

Eat fewer processed and cured meats (like ham, bacon, sausage, frankfurters, and luncheon meats high in saturated fats, sodium, and artificial preservatives).

Select lean cuts such as eye round, sirloin tips, shoulder, chuck, flank, tenderloin, and remove all visible fat before preparing.

Eat poultry (white meat without the skin) which has less saturated fat and fewer calories than beef or pork.

Eat fish which is low in fat. However, tuna, salmon, and sardines canned in oil contain more fat and less protein, so purchase them canned in water.

Nuts and seeds are rich sources of vegetable protein but also contain a high concentration of calories and fat (mainly the "good" polyunsaturated kind). Sunflower seeds, sesame seeds, walnuts, almonds, and peanuts are the best sources.

Although eggs are an excellent source of high quality protein, the yolks contain a concentrated source of fat and cholesterol. Limit intake to three or four eggs a week, or eat only the whites of the egg.

DAIRY PRODUCTS

Eat reduced- or non-fat dairy products such as skimmed milk, low-fat cottage cheese, plain yogurt, and low-fat cheeses. Reduce the amount of cream, ice cream (ice milk has about half the fat of ice cream), whole milk, whipped cream, and cream cheese. These products contain excess fat and calories.

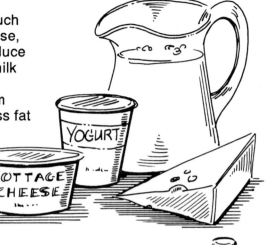

FATS AND OILS

Use more polyunsaturated vegetable oils such as safflower, corn, and sunflower.

Margarines high in polyunsaturates (usually the softer kind) are preferred.

Avoid hydrogenated fats (the process that makes fats more saturated).

Avoid palm oil and coconut oil, which are also high in saturated fat.

FRUITS AND VEGETABLES

Eat raw fruits and vegetables daily. Many vitamins and minerals are destroyed in the cooking process.

Eat dried peas and beans, which in their natural state are excellent low-fat sources of protein.

BREADS AND CEREALS

Eat whole grain breads and cereals rather than refined ones. During the refining process, essential "B" vitamins and minerals are removed along with the bran (the outer layer of wheat kernel). Vitamin E is also lost when the wheat germ is expelled. Enriched breads and cereals replace many (but not all) of the lost nutrients.

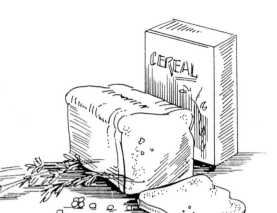

MISCELLANEOUS TIPS

Avoid eating large meals. A large meal elevates blood sugars and fatty acids. This extra food will usually be stored as fat in your body. Eat small meals at more frequent intervals throughout the day.

Foods that are cooked, stored in the refrigerator (or freezer), and then reheated later lose many of their vitamins.

Eat more slowly and chew your food completely. Fast eating encourages overeating.

Drink an average of 8 to 10 glasses of water a day (along with other fluids).

Avoid overusing the salt shaker.

Limit consumption of cookies, cakes, and candies; they contain excessive amounts of sugar and fat.

Read the label panels of foods to evaluate the nutrient content and look for hidden ingredients.

Include more fiber in your diet. The typical American diet is too high in calories, sugars, fats, and sodium.

Drink no more than two cups of coffee a day to avoid symptoms of anxiety such as nervousness, irritability, increased blood pressure, muscle tension, and difficulty sleeping.

Avoid skipping meals (especially breakfast). Many times when meals are skipped people more than make up for it at another meal. Substitute fruits for desserts.

If you are going to drink, drink moderate amounts of alcohol.

SPECIAL FOCUS: WEIGHT MANAGEMENT

The technical cause of excess weight and obesity is an energy imbalance in the body. Improper diet, overeating, hormonal disturbances, psychological factors, and physical inactivity may create a positive energy imbalance, resulting in a gain of weight. It should be noted that only a small percentage of cases of obesity are actually attributable to hormonal disorders. There is a strong genetic predisposition for children to be obese if one or both parents are obese. This does not compensate for the effect of poor eating habits and other environmental influences, such as inactivity.

The primary emphasis in any weight management program should be on combining diet and exercise. Not only will this type of program assist in the loss of weight, but the specific weight that will be lost will be the unwanted fat pounds. A combination of long duration, low-intensity aerobic exercise and resistance exercise will benefit you most. The low-intensity aerobic exercise will stimulate the release of hormones that increase the mobilization of fatty acids from fat deposit storage. Resistance exercise will increase your lean muscle tissue mass and contribute to caloric consumption.

Eat at least 1000 calories per day, which include an ample amount of complex carbohydrates, to get enough nutrient dense foods to supply basic bodily needs. Avoid succumbing to those well-advertised, fad diets. Many of these programs ignore sound nutritional guidelines and result predominantly in water loss and a health risk to the dieter. Also, many people fast in order to lose weight. This subjects the body to a condition that actually increases the activity of fat depositing enzymes. Your body is reacting to what it perceives as starvation conditions and tries to protect itself from not being supplied the necessary foodstuffs. Thus, larger amounts of carbohydrates and proteins will be converted and stored as fats. Nutrition experts recommend at least three and as many as six smaller meals a day. Finally, if you are aware that you have some type of eating behavior disorder, seek some professional help.

Here is an aerobic exercise prescription to promote weight loss.

1) Mode: any aerobic exercise that you enjoy including walking, running, swimming, cycling, aerobic dance, etc.
2) Intensity: 60% to 70% of your personalized target zone
3) Duration: 30 to 60 minutes
4) Frequency: 5 to 7 times a week
5) Length of program: until desired goals are obtained

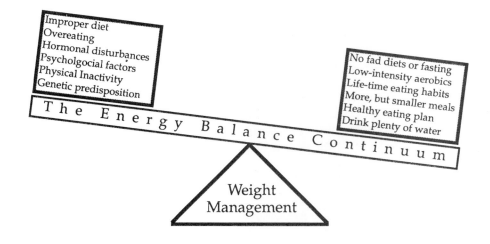

Improper diet
Overeating
Hormonal disturbances
Psycholgocial factors
Physical Inactivity
Genetic predisposition

No fad diets or fasting
Low-intensity aerobics
Life-time eating habits
More, but smaller meals
Healthy eating plan
Drink plenty of water

The Energy Balance Continuum

Weight Management

STRESS

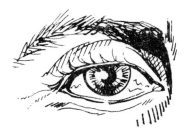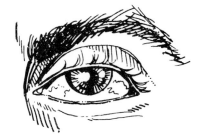

Stress is an inevitable part of living. Life does have its ups and downs. Excessive stress and burnout can have emotional consequences.

One of the main causes of stress is a sudden, drastic, unwanted change: personal loss in the family, a job crisis, injury or illness, financial problems, and emotional problems all fall into this category. The tension from stress often leads to that worried, uptight sensation we call anxiety—you feel angered or frustrated. If these feelings continue to obstruct your ability to enjoy life, physical ailments such as ulcers and high blood pressure may result.

Being "stressed-out" may even lead to depression. Do you recognize the symptoms? Restlessness, feelings of inadequacy and insecurity, inability to concentrate, sleeplessness, and lack of interest in food, life and social interaction are all signs of depression. **You _can_ beat it! You _can_ take charge!**

Follow these guidelines:

1) Talk over your problems with a close friend or seek professional advice. You need to express your feelings!
2) See a physician if you have any physical ailments.
3) Do vigorous exercise regularly to vent anxiety and to combat depression.
4) Don't overload yourself. Set practical goals you can reach successfully and timetables you can meet.
5) Learn to relax. You need some peace and quiet each day just for **you!**
6) Organize your work and personal affairs. This will give you more efficient use of your time and will rid your life of clutter.
7) Take short breaks or a vacation. Time out will give you a better perspective.
8) Look ahead. Sometimes you can anticipate a job slump, a budding problem, financial difficulties, etc. and be prepared.
9) Stay away from drugs and alcohol—they are just temporary relievers of tension, not cures for problems.
10) Improve your eating habits and your diet. Don't skip meals because you are too busy.

STRESS RELEASE BREATHING INTERVENTION:

Here's a simple breathing drill you can do anytime to help lesson the effects of stress. Sit very comfortably and focus on relaxing your muscles in your body, especially those that are tensing up. Keep your breathing very slow and controlled. As you inhale say to yourself, "I am," and as you exhale say to yourself, "relaxed." continue for 3 to 5 minutes.

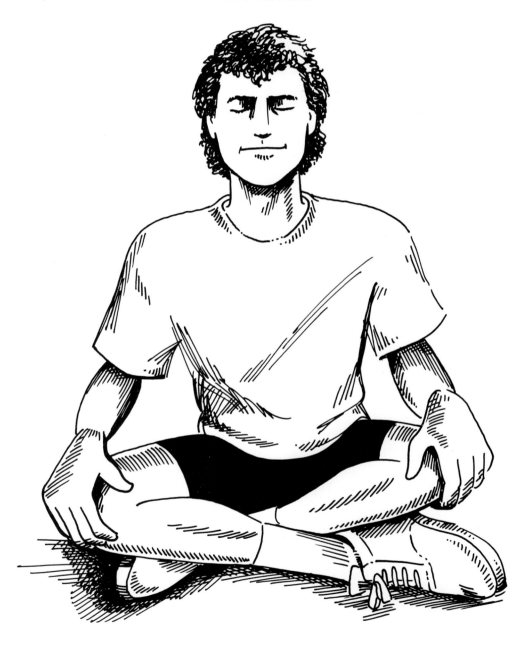

FITNESS GEAR AND WHERE TO TRAIN

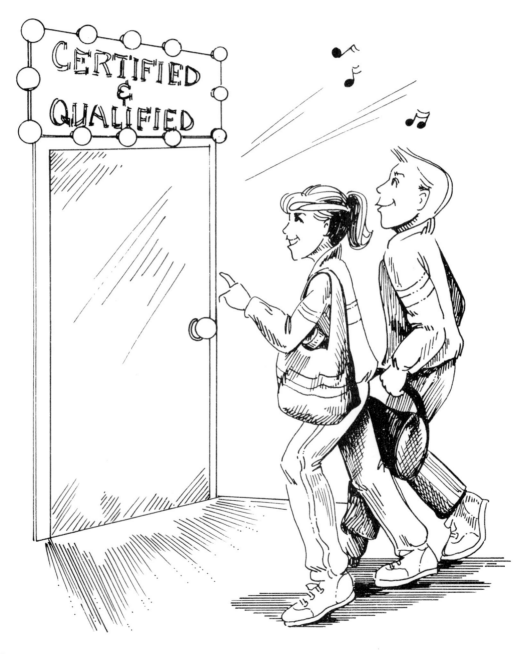

IN SEARCH OF THE PERFECT AEROBIC SHOE

The most important investment you can make for aerobics is your shoe. You want a shoe with flexibility, that supports your arches, cushions your heels, adds extra impact absorption at the balls of your feet, and that fits well. Here's what to check out:

The outersole should be flexible, yet durable.

The midsole (between the outer and inner sole) should provide good stability and cushioning to absorb shock, yet allow for foot flexibility.

The innersole: A high-shock-absorbent material such as Sorbothane or Spenco is recommended. If the shoe you like doesn't have this, purchase an innersole separately.

The toe area: This is the one place on the shoe where roominess counts. When you exercise, your foot swells. Allow for it. Can you wiggle your toes?

Forefoot cushion: The greatest amount of force the foot must absorb is just behind the ball of the foot. There must be good cushioning here.

Forefoot flexibility: The shoe should bend (as the foot does) at the ball of the foot. Too stiff a forefoot will cause lower leg discomfort. This area needs to be flexible yet stable.

Arch support: Make sure the arch provides comfortable support.

The heel counter: This should be an inflexible material surrounding the heel area, holding it in place. The more it prevents excessive rolling and twisting, the better it is.

The shoe heel: Look for an outer heel that makes a flush contact with the ground. If the inner heel height is too low, it will cause an excessive pull on the calf and Achilles tendon. The heel should provide good cushion without being too hard or too soft. Shoes are now designed in high top ankle support. These help out a lot.

Comfort: Try them on in the store and move around for 10 minutes. Don't purchase if they feel uncomfortable. Also, since your feet swell during the day, it is best to purchase shoes in the afternoon or evening.

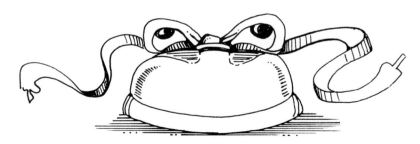

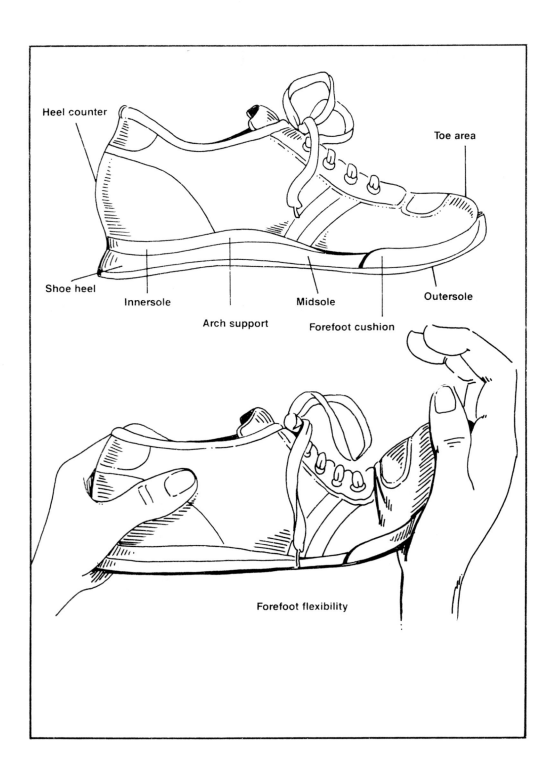

Heel counter

Toe area

Shoe heel

Innersole

Arch support

Midsole

Forefoot cushion

Outersole

Forefoot flexibility

58

HOW TO JOIN A HEALTH CLUB

Try to visit the prospective health club during the time you would be using the facility. Shop around, using the following as a helpful checklist:

1) Is the location convenient to your home, work, or school?
2) Is it a workout gym, a social club, a co-ed facility, or a fitness center for families? What are you looking for?
3) Does the facility look clean, organized, seasonally air-controlled, and suitably lighted? Specifically check out the locker room and showers for cleanliness!
4) What facilities should you look for?
   a. Well-equipped exercise rooms with top equipment. Are there enough weight-resistive machines, stationary bikes, treadmills, rowing machines, free weights, and space to accommodate the members?
   b. Anaerobic exercise room with a proper floor. Does it have a floating wood design or is it carpet, wood, or linoleum over cement (which is much more unsafe)? Does it have enough space for the class sizes? Is it air conditioned?

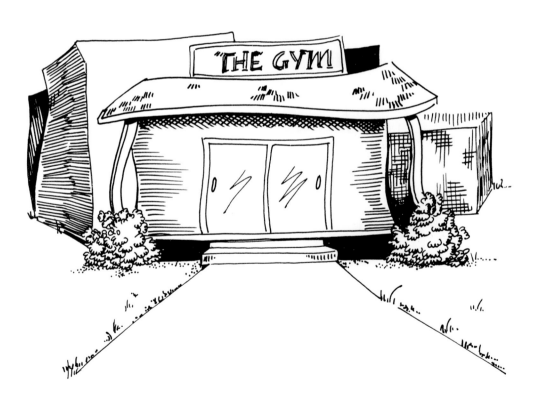

c. Accessible racquetball or squash courts. What is the court reservation procedure? (If you have to reserve over 48 hours in advance you know that they are getting heavy use.) Do the court floors and walls look very marked up? Do you have to pay for court time?

d. Well-maintained pool. Is it heated year-round? Is the size suitable to your needs?

e. Available track facilities. Is there an indoor or outdoor track?

f. Relaxing spa facilities. Is there a whirlpool, sauna, steam room, massage room, and cold plunge?

g. Well-kept locker room. Do you get a locker and key every time you use the facility? Or do you bring your own lock or rent out the locker? Does the club provide towels, soap, shampoo, hair dryers, and other grooming amenities?

5) What kind of staff does it have? Are there any trained personnel in physical education, exercise physiology, nutrition, or sports medicine? Does the staff have a professional, friendly, and helpful attitude?

6) What type of programs do they run? Are there enough classes in a variety of workouts? Are there additional fees? Can you take a class any time you wish?

7) Do the club hours fit your needs?

8) **Examine the fees carefully!**

a. Are they affordable? Is there a payment plan?

b. Is there an initiation fee? Is it refundable? Is this a one-time charge or yearly charge? Are there any monthly dues in addition? How much?

c. Be leery of contracts and "too good to be true" promotionals. Read all the small print before you sign.

d. Be wary of "lifetime" memberships—is it **your** lifetime or the **club's**?

e. What are the cancellation policies? Must you sell your membership? Do you get a prorated refund?

9) Does the club allow you to put your membership on hold for a short period (such as for a vacation) without having to pay the monthly dues?

10) How much does it cost to bring a guest to the club? Does the club give out guest passes?

CREATING A HOME GYM

You don't have to be rich to create a convenient home gym. Even if you belong to a club or studio, your schedule or occasional desire for workout privacy may warrant the purchase of home exercise equipment. Here are some tips to get you started:

1) Make sure you have enough space. A wall mirror helps you view your exercise technique and serves as a great motivator. Music helps too!
2) Make sure the lighting and air ventilation are adequate.
3) Before purchasing any equipment, identify your fitness needs. Do you want a jump rope, treadmill, stationary cycle, or rowing machine for cardiorespiratory fitness? Do you want equipment for specific exercises for your abdominals, legs, and buttocks? Having identified your fitness needs will prevent you from purchasing equipment of no value to you.
4) Look for equipment which features effective safety measures and provides progressive exercise guidelines.
5) Shop around. It's amazing how the cost of the same equipment varies from store to store! Examine the warranty and service agreements closely.
6) Watch out for attractive, shiny, lightweight equipment that lacks durability and stability.
7) Try the equipment out. Not all equipment feels the same. With mail order equipment, review the return policies and procedures carefully before purchasing. Are the shipping charges reasonable?
8) Build your exercise area to fit your program. Buy a little at a time and add as you see fit.
9) Stay away from products that guarantee phenomenal results in a short time.
10) When purchasing equipment on sale, see if the product is being discontinued. If it is, there may be a newer, better style available at the same price.
11) For display purposes, store equipment is usually free-standing and movable. Check to see which products need to be firmly secured to a wall or floor, and how they need to be secured.

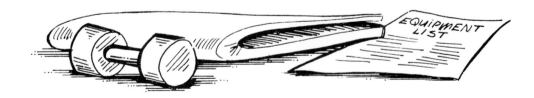

FINDING THE RIGHT INSTRUCTOR

All instructors have their own teaching styles and classes have their own special characteristics. Here's what to look for in an instructor and class to make sure it meets your needs:

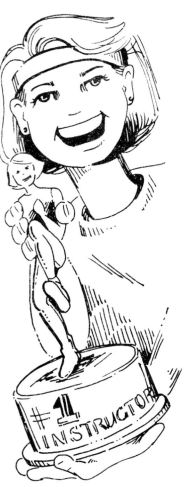

1) Take a trial class or observe the instructor and class during the time you would normally attend.
2) Look for **quality** and not **quantity.** Just because a class does numerous repetitions or the instructor is "tuff" doesn't mean it's a good class.
3) Does the instructor make an effort to teach, correct, explain, and give clear directions? Can you hear the verbal instructions? Does the instructor modify exercises for the students who have special needs?
4) If there is a mirror, does the instructor face it throughout most of the class? Mirrors are wonderful instructional aids, but direct eye contact is one of the most effective means of communication and interaction.
5) Look for a well-rounded workout: a thorough warm-up, a gradually building aerobic section, a winding down of the aerobics, a complete body firming section, and a cool-down stretching segment.
6) Does the workout seem to flow smoothly from one section to the next?
7) Is the class easy to follow? Could you see the instructor easily or was it too crowded?

8) Does the instructor inspire and motivate you? Did you enjoy the workout?
9) Was the workout challenging enough for you? Does the club or studio offer a variety of different levels and styles of classes?
10) Did you feel comfortable with the class atmosphere?
11) Could you hear the music? Was it too loud?
12) What training, credentials, and education does the instructor have? The credibility of an instructor who boasts of "being certified" cannot always be substantiated. Inquire about any specific training, experience, and education the instructor has had.
13) Does the class follow a prescribed exercise program? The American College of Sports Medicine recommends three to five times a week of aerobic activity, between 15 and 60 minutes, at 55 percent to 90 percent of your maximum heart rate range.
14) Is there any type of medical screening for participants prior to participation?
15) Is the cost of the class or program within your budget?
16) Is the class in a convenient location?

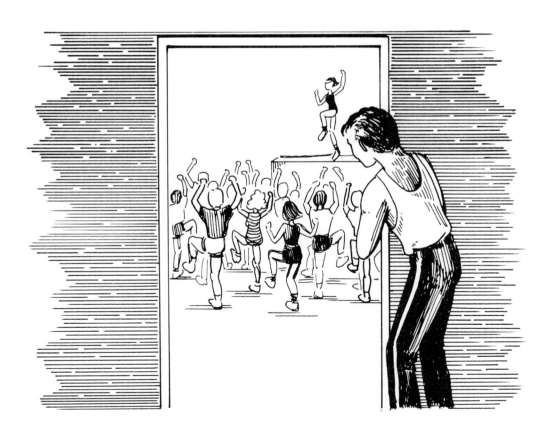

LET'S WORK OUT

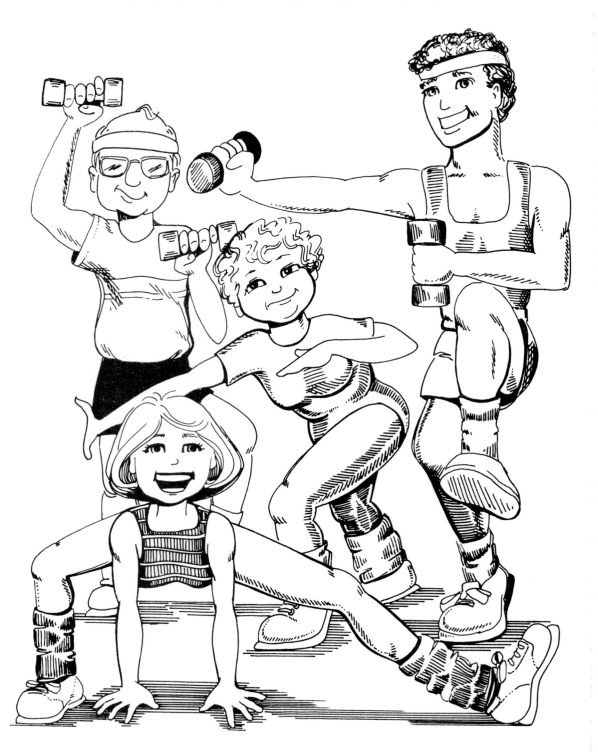

WARM UP FIRST

Let's get ready for the movement to follow and prevent any injuries!

WARM-UP DO'S AND DON'TS:
DO MOVE SLOWLY AND RHYTHMICALLY.
DO FOCUS ON FULL-BODY EXTENSION.
DO PERFORM ALL WARM-UP EXERCISES
   ON BOTH SIDES.
DO HOLD WARM-UP FLOOR STRETCHES
   FROM 15 TO 30 SECONDS.
DON'T BOUNCE, JERK, OR FORCE
   POSITIONS.
DON'T "LOCK" YOUR JOINTS.

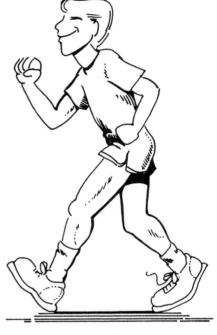

FIRST OFF: ACTIVE START
   Begin with three to five minutes of **easy** aerobics, brisk walking, or cycling to elevate the body temperature, stimulate circulation to the muscles, and loosen up the joints to prepare them for more strenuous exercise.
   Then, try this series of warm-up exercises:

HEAD (For neck)
   ACTION: Take head from one side, forward, and around to other side. Reverse. Also, turn head from side to side.
   TIPS: avoid taking the head to a straight back position. Make sure these movements are performed slowly.

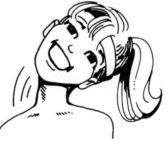

SHOULDER ROLLS (For shoulders)
  ACTION: Smooth circles with shoulders
  (arms down at side).
  TIPS: Circle in both directions.

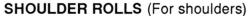

TORSO SIDE STRETCH (For side and hips)
  ACTION: Reach one arm over your head and
  stretch your torso sideways. Stretch other
  side. Keep the knees slightly bent.
  TIPS: Be sure to face forward so you don't
  twist as you stretch. Support yourself with
  your extended arm on the thigh to avoid spinal
  stress.

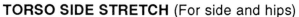

TORSO TWIST (For spine)
  ACTION: Twist gently and rhythmically from
  the waist.
  TIPS: Keep your knees slightly bent and
  control the movement.

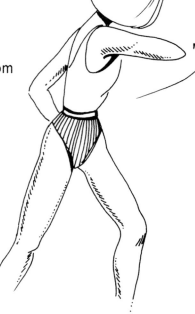

BENT-LEG BODY CIRCLE

(For hips, spine, back of the legs)
ACTION: The arms reach in a continuous circle from overhead, to the side, floor, and back up.
TIPS: Bend the knees! And keep the head up.

LUNGE STRETCH: HIGH AND LOW

(For thighs and lower leg)
ACTION: Bend front knee and keep back leg straight. **HIGH LUNGE:** Stretch the Achilles tendon and calf by gently bending and straightening the back leg. **LOW LUNGE:** Stretch the hips down into the floor. Other side.
TIPS: Keep the front knee over the ankle and the toes pointing forward.

UPPER SPINE/SHOULDER STRETCH

ACTION: Place hands on thighs above knees. Keep your knees bent. Press one shoulder down and allow the trunk and head to rotate, stretching the upper back, shoulder, and neck. To other side.
TIPS: Always keep your knees slightly bent and do not bend over too far forward.

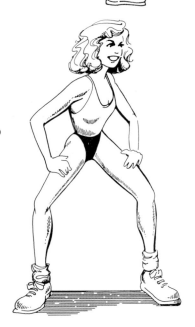

AEROBICS: THE MAIN EVENT

Here are some aerobic dance steps you can perform to lively music. Start gradually at a brisk walking pace, increase your intensity into your target zone, and then wind back down to a brisk walk. To improve your aerobic efficiency, build up to 20 continuous minutes, three to five times a week. Be creative and "choreograph" your own routines! You can create variety by using various arm positions, lifting your legs to different heights, adding a clap, and traveling in a circle or in different directions. Also, all aerobic skills can be modified by just bending and lifting the legs without "bouncing" on the floor. This is called "low-impact" aerobics. A combination of "low-impact" with "impact" aerobics is recommended to reduce the potential of overuse injuries on the body's lower extremities.

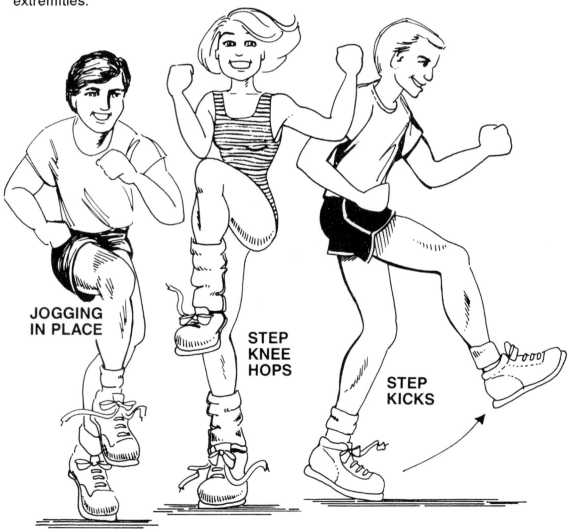

JOGGING
IN PLACE

STEP
KNEE
HOPS

STEP
KICKS

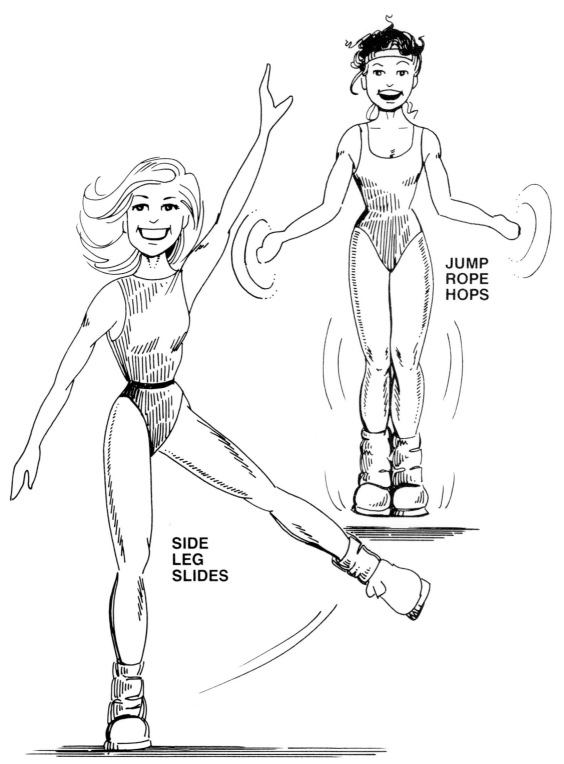

JUMP
ROPE
HOPS

SIDE
LEG
SLIDES

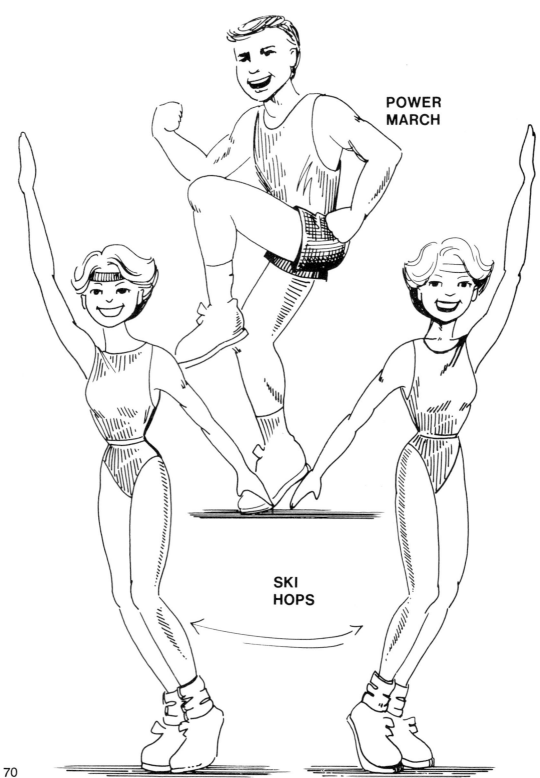

POWER
MARCH

SKI
HOPS

70

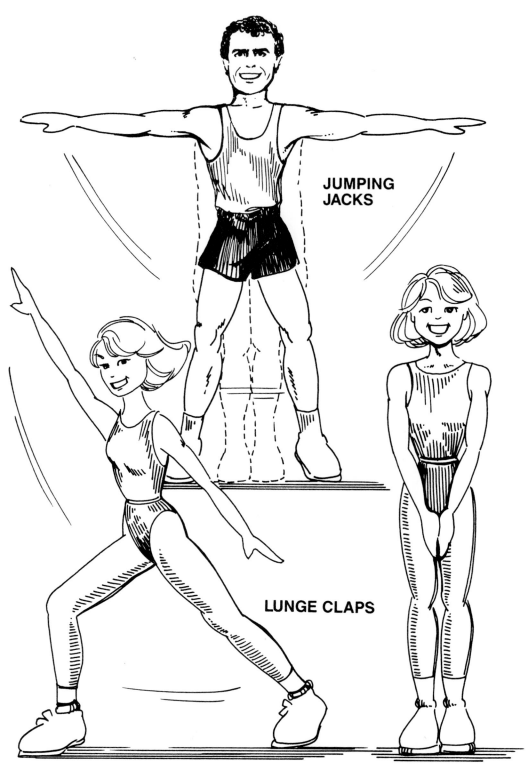

JUMPING
JACKS

LUNGE CLAPS

71

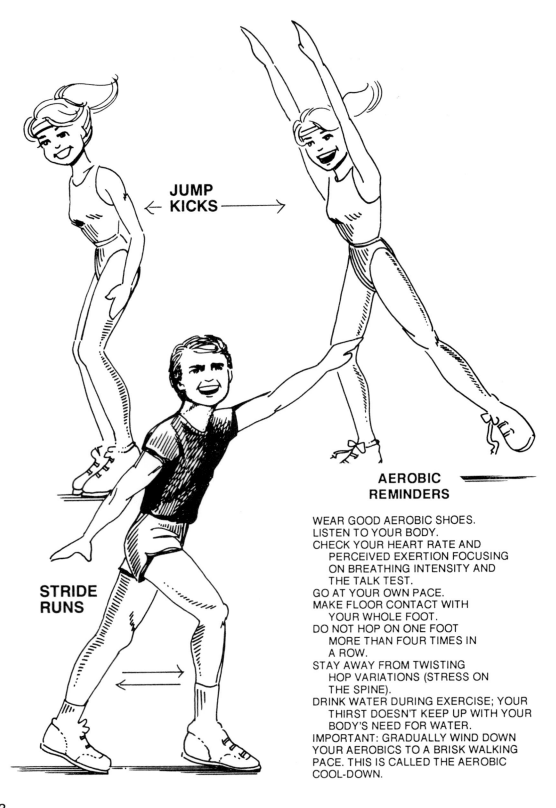

JUMP ← KICKS →

STRIDE RUNS

AEROBIC REMINDERS

WEAR GOOD AEROBIC SHOES.
LISTEN TO YOUR BODY.
CHECK YOUR HEART RATE AND
  PERCEIVED EXERTION FOCUSING
  ON BREATHING INTENSITY AND
  THE TALK TEST.
GO AT YOUR OWN PACE.
MAKE FLOOR CONTACT WITH
  YOUR WHOLE FOOT.
DO NOT HOP ON ONE FOOT
  MORE THAN FOUR TIMES IN
  A ROW.
STAY AWAY FROM TWISTING
  HOP VARIATIONS (STRESS ON
  THE SPINE).
DRINK WATER DURING EXERCISE; YOUR
  THIRST DOESN'T KEEP UP WITH YOUR
  BODY'S NEED FOR WATER.
IMPORTANT: GRADUALLY WIND DOWN
YOUR AEROBICS TO A BRISK WALKING
PACE. THIS IS CALLED THE AEROBIC
COOL-DOWN.

STEPPING INTO THE 90'S

Within the last few years, stair climbing has gained incredible popularity. In athletic clubs and schools around the country, members are lining up to go through their workout on new, computerized stair systems that promote improvements in cardiorespiratory endurance, fat loss, and leg and buttocks strength development. This fast rise to popularity can be attributed in part to the unintimidating, user-friendly, but challenging nature of these high-tech stepping machines. Also, the concept of cross-training, which integrates different fitness activities into a total-body fitness program, has certainly been influential to the remarkable acceptance of stair stepping. More recently, the growth of bench stepping for class and home use has arrived. Fitness professionals, wanting to expand upon traditional aerobic workouts, have begun to incorporate various bench stepping combinations into complete workouts.

Bench stepping can best be described as a low-impact activity capable of providing high-intensity aerobic conditioning for the participant. The workout can be as challenging as vigorous jogging and yet produce impact forces as safe as walking. The feeling of this activity is very similar to the workout you get from climbing stairs. The cadence of the stepping is slower than the movement tempos you would use in an aerobic class (approximately 118 to 126 beats per minutes), because of the greater ranges of motion offered by the platform and because of a concern for safety.

Benches range in height from 4 inches to 12 inches high and have a stepping surface of 14 inches wide and up to 4 feet long. It is recommended that you begin gradually, using a lower height box, and progressively increase towards taller boxes as you become more capable of handling demanding stepping heights. The bench workout is an excellent supplement to your favorite aerobic program, allowing you to alternate workouts from day to day if you so choose.

I have presented the basic steps and patterns for you to learn on your step. Treat this workout like any other workout. You need to warm-up your body the same as prescribed in the warm-up section. Devote a little more time to warm-up the calves for a step training workout. Accompany this workout with specific body sculpturing exercises of your choice, and don't forget your cool-down stretches at the end of the workout. Each step is most easily categorized by the direction in which the body faces the platform. The specific directions include:

a) From the front
b) From the side
c) From a straddle stand
d) From the top
e) From the end

Each step is further classified as either a basic or single lead step where the same foot leads every cycle, or as an alternating step where the lead step alternates every four counts. When doing a single lead step, a good rule to follow is to lead with the same leg for no more than 1 minute before changing to the other foot. When doing an alternating lead step, a good rule to follow is to continue the step for no longer than 2 minutes. What about arm choreography? Focus on learning the basic steps at first. Arm choreography will come naturally as you become more comfortable with your stepping patterns.

Here are some basic moves to get you stepping.

1. **BASIC STEP:**
   a) Directional approach: From the front
   b) Performance: Right foot up, left foot up, right foot down, left foot down, and continue. (Do on both sides)
   c) Pattern: Up, up, down, down

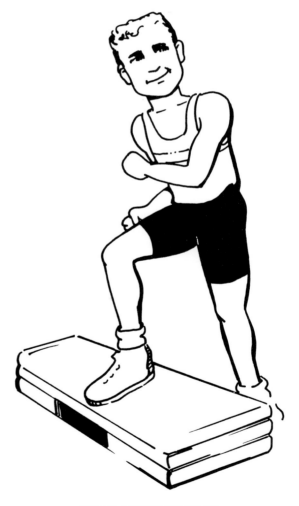

FROM THE FRONT

2. **ALTERNATING BASIC STEP:**
   a) Directional approach: From the front
   b) Performance: Right foot up, left foot up, right foot down, left foot down (tap), switch lead to left foot up, right foot up, left foot down, right foot down (tap) switch lead, and continue
   c) Pattern: Up, up, down, tap up, up, down, tap
3. **BASIC V-STEP:**
   a) Directional approach: From the front
   b) Performance: right foot up and out, left foot up and out, right foot down, left foot down, and continue. (Do on both sides)
      • Performance Tip: Step with a wide V pattern by opening the legs on top of the platform and bringing them together on the floor.
   c) Pattern: Up, up, down, down
   d) Variation: Can also do with an alternating basic step pattern

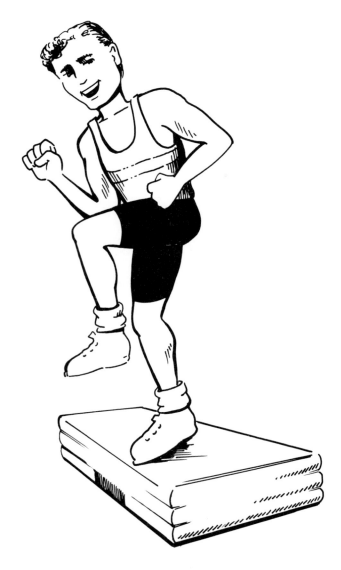

STEP KNEE

4. **ALTERNATING KNEE-UP STEP:**
   a) Directional approach: From the front
   b) Performance: Right foot up, left knee up, left foot down, right foot down.
      Left foot up, right knee up, right foot down, right foot down. continue pattern.
   c) Pattern: Up, knee, down, down; up other knee, down, down

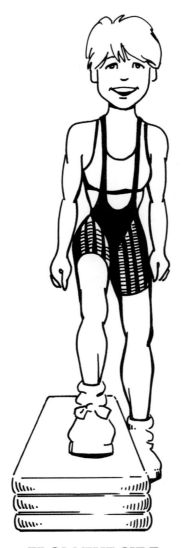

FROM THE SIDE

5. **ACROSS THE TOP STEP:**
   a) Directional approach: From the side
   b) Performance: right foot up, left foot up, right foot down, left foot down (tap), switch to left foot up, right foot up, left foot down, right foot down (tap). Continue the alternating across the top pattern.
   c) Pattern: up, across, down, tap; up, across, down, tap

6. **STRADDLE DOWN STEP:**
   a) Directional approach: From the top
   b) Performance: Right foot down on side of platform, left foot down on side of platform, right foot up, left foot up. (Do on both sides)
   c) Pattern: down, down, up, up
   d) Variation: Can also do with an alternating step pattern

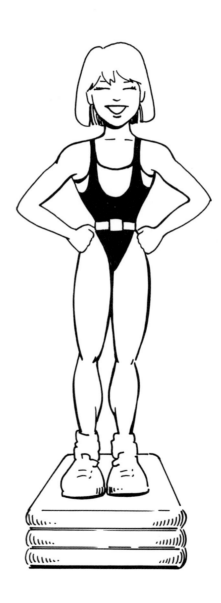

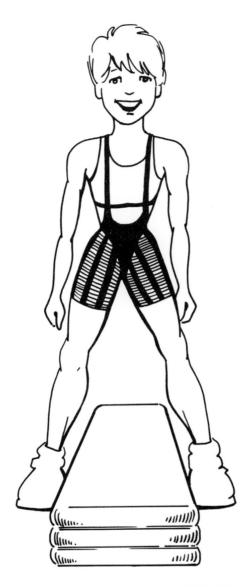

FROM A STRADDLE STAND

7. **STRADDLE UP STEP:**
   a) Directional approach: From a straddle stand
   b) Performance: right foot up, left foot up, right foot down, left foot down. (Do on both sides)
   c) Pattern: Up, up, down, down
   d) Variation: Can also do with an alternating step pattern

79

8. **ALTERNATING STRADDLE KNEE LIFT STEP:**
   a) Directional approach: From a straddle stand
   b) Performance: Right foot up, left knee lift, left foot down to floor, right foot down to floor. Left foot up, right knee lift, right knee down to floor, left foot down to floor. Continue the alternating knee lift pattern.
   c) Pattern: Up, knee lift, down, down; Up, knee lift, down, down
9. **ALTERNATING SIDE LUNGE STEP:**
   a) Directional approach: From the top
   b) Performance: Right foot down and out, right foot on top of platform; left foot down and out, left foot on top of platform. Continue alternating from side to side.
   c) Pattern: Lunge out, up, lunge out, up

10. **FROM THE END STEP:**
   a)   Directional approach: From the end
   b)   Performance: Use the end of the platform to combine several of the steps introduced above for variety.

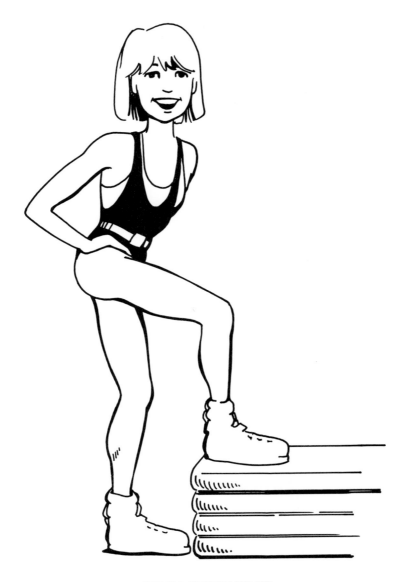

FROM THE END

STEPPING SAFETY TO SUCCESS:

1) Make sure you step entirely on the top part of the platform with each step, not allowing any part of your foot to hang over the edge.

2) Start with a 4" or 6" height. Don't rush to raise the height of the bench. Most people find the 8" height to provide a satisfactory workout. The recommendation to avoid flexing the knee more than 90 degrees with your step height is a conservative guideline that is easy to follow.

3) Adding hand-held weights (up to 3 lbs.) Changes your arm choreography to slow, controlled, non-rotational, shorter-lever movements.

4) Stop stepping and march in place on the ground whenever you want to lower the intensity.

5) Be careful not to step too far back off the platform. This causes the body to lean slightly forward, placing extra stress on the Achilles tendon and calf.

6) Use a good cross-training shoe or aerobic shoe for your workout. The tread on some running shoes does not provide suitable freedom of movement and support on some platforms.

7) Step onto and off of the platform. Avoid pounding your feet on the ground and platform. Also, try not to step with a bounce, this causes you to remain on the balls of your feet.

8) Remember not to lock your knees on the descending phase of the step pattern.

9) Avoid any movements that travel forward and down off the bench.

10) Drink plenty of water as you tend to sweat a little more with step training.

11) Be aware of the potential for overuse injury syndrome. Many people will enjoy the variety and uniqueness of step training so much that they will discontinue their other physical activities. Doing a variety of exercise programs lessens the stress on many specific body parts, and still allows you to place a lot of demands on your body.

12) If you feel any discomfort underneath or around the knee you need to stop. See your health practitioner. Bench stepping may not be the best activity for you.

13) Always watch your platform when stepping.

14) As you step, avoid unnecessary forward bending at the hips. This may put too much stress on your back.

15) Be careful of overusing the lunge skills. They can cause you to lean too far forward, stressing your lower back, and they can place extra joint trauma on the lower leg with ground impact.

THE CHEST, SHOULDER, AND ARM DEVELOPERS

PERFORM 10 TO 30 REPETITIONS OF EACH EXERCISE.

MODIFIED OR REGULAR PUSH-UPS (Chest, shoulders, and arms)
   ACTION: Lower torso all the way to the floor and up.
   TIPS: Keep the back straight.

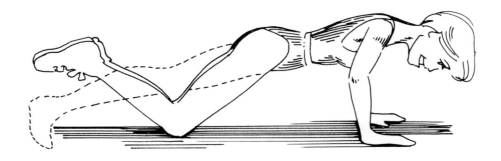

WIDE-ARM PUSH-UPS (Chest and arms)
   ACTION: Same as push-up with arms placed beyond shoulder width.
Open legs to a straddle position.
   TIPS: Make sure fingers are pointed away from body.

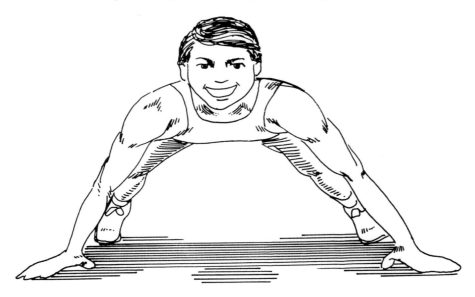

PIKE PUSH-UPS (Shoulders and triceps—back of the arms)
   ACTION: A push-up with hips up and hands closer to feet. Legs together or open to a straddle.
   TIPS: Placing the hands closer together is more challenging.

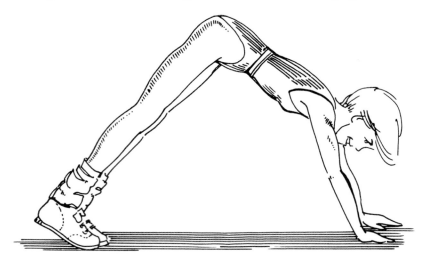

DIPS (Shoulders, chest and triceps)
   ACTION: With hands by side on chair or floor, bend and extend arms.
   TIPS: Hands should face forward. Keep legs extended when using chair.

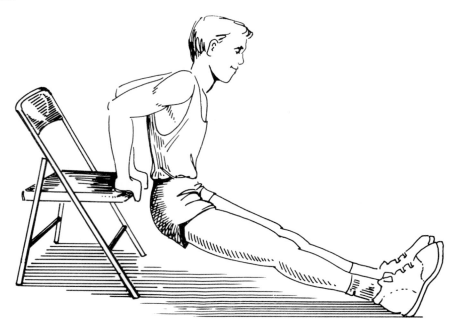

CHEST/ELBOW SQUEEZE (Chest and biceps—front of arms)
  ACTION: Lift arms in front of chest, bend arms to 45 degrees and squeeze elbows, forearms, and wrists together.
  TIPS: Hold each squeeze for at least six seconds.
  VARIATION: Lift the elbows and arms up and down as they are contracting against each other.

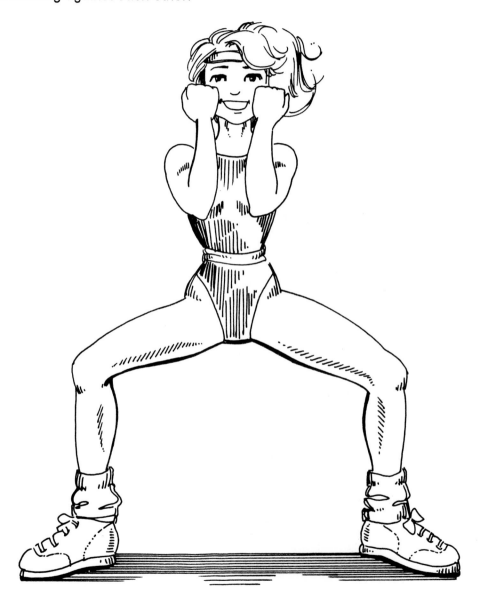

FOR THE ABDOMINALS:
THE FABULOUS FIVE

PERFORM 15 TO 40 REPETITIONS OF EACH EXERCISE.

REGULAR CRUNCH (Abdominals)
ACTION: Lift the back and shoulders off the floor. Push the small of the back against the floor. Rotate pelvis so buttocks are slightly off floor.
TIPS: Feet are on the floor approximately six inches from the buttocks. Hands may support the head at the base of the neck or lie across the chest. Focus on the ceiling.
VARIATION: Squeeze your knees together for inner thigh work as well.

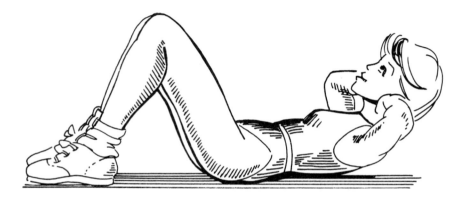

TWISTING CRUNCH (Abdominals and obliques—sides)
ACTION: Alternate shoulders as you lift your upper back off the floor.
TIPS: Vary your technique by either lifting first and then twisting or by twisting first and then lifting.

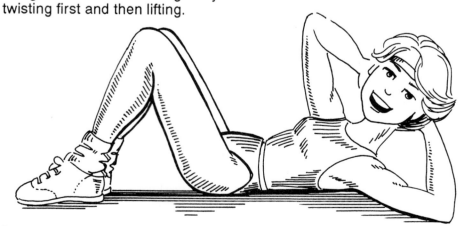

REVERSE CRUNCH (Lower abdominals)
  ACTION: Slowly lift buttocks off the ground a couple of inches.
  TIPS: Keep the knees bent.
  VARIATION: Bring chest towards knee
  (as you lift the buttocks) for an even
  more challenging crunch. Press the heels
  into the buttocks to relax your hip
  flexors and work the abdominals more.

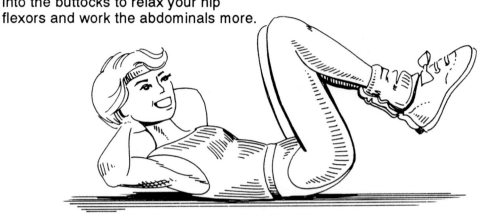

ROPE PULL CRUNCH (Abdominals and obliques)
  ACTION: Lift shoulder blades off the floor and alternate
  reaching the arms (as if pulling a rope).
  TIPS: Make sure the small of the back
  is pressed into floor.

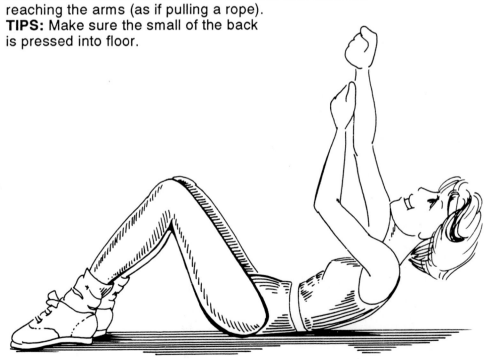

THE ALL-AROUND CRUNCH (Abdominals and obliques)
ACTION: Alternate with a twisting crunch to one side, a regular crunch straight up, and a twisting crunch to the other side.

TIPS: Lift the legs so the thighs are perpendicular to the floor and bent at the knees. You may wish to place your feet on a chair.

VARIATION: Randomly mix the pattern of the side, up, other side to surprise your abdominal muscles—they have to work harder!

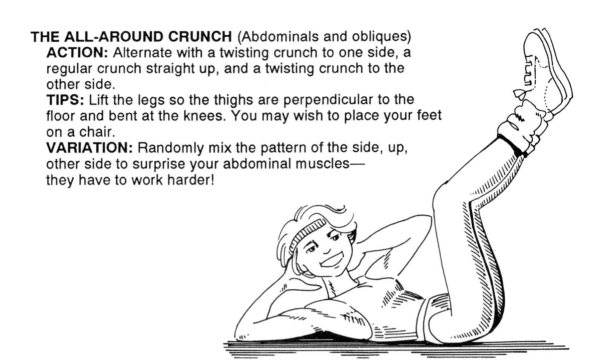

BACK EXTENSION (After working the abdominal muscles, it is correct to work the opposite muscle group: the lower back.)
ACTION: Slowly lift the head, shoulders, and chest off the floor from the prone position. The arms may help with the lift, remain at the sides, or be held close to the shoulders.

TIPS: Keep the feet on the floor to protect the spine. Stretch up and out.

GREATER ABDOMINAL WORK OPTIONS:
Vary your tempo of performance so your body does not rely on momentum.

Rotate the pelvis so the buttocks come slightly off the floor.

Use a weight (two to ten pounds) behind the head or across the chest.

Try to keep shoulders from touching all the way on the floor when coming down each time.

OUTER THIGH, HIPS, AND BUTTOCKS

These body parts are best worked **together!** As you become competent, you need to overload. Wear leg weights or use elastic resistance (such as a strong rubber band).

PERFORM 15 TO 30 REPETITIONS OF EACH EXERCISE.

OUTER LEG LIFTS (Outer thigh and hip)
    ACTION: On your side with your head supported by your arm (elbow on the ground), bottom knee bent for balance. Lift the top leg up and down, keeping the foot parallel to the floor.
    TIPS: Make sure the top hip is directly above the bottom hip.
Bring the bottom knee forward to release any tension on the spine. Both knees are facing forward.
    VARIATION: May also do with torso on floor.

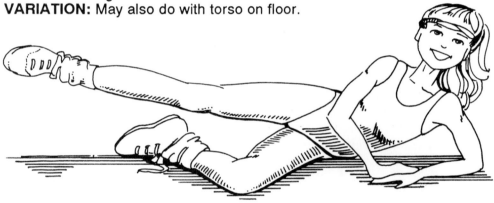

SIDE LEG CIRCLES (Outer thigh and hip)
    ACTION: Same position as outer leg lift.
Make slow circles in both directions with the top leg.
    TIPS: Vary the size of your circles.

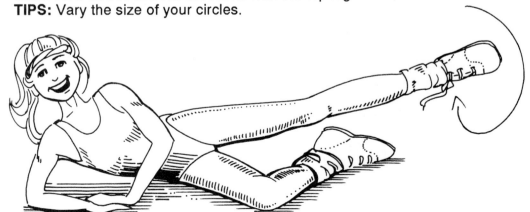

FORWARD SIDE LEG LIFTS (Outer thigh and hip)

ACTION: Same position, but bring your top leg forward about 45 degrees. Now perform outer leg lift in this position.

TIPS: Do not bring your leg so far forward that it places your body in a letter "T." This can stress the hip joint.

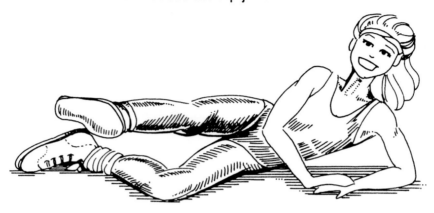

PRONE LEG LIFTS (Buttocks)

ACTION: Assume a prone position on your side and your stomach— half on each. Lift the leg of the elevated hip up and down slowly. Your top leg crosses over the bottom leg as it lowers.

TIPS: Keep your body straight and support yourself with your arms. Keep your head on the floor. This position takes pressure off your lower back by keeping it from sagging. Keep toes of lifting leg pointed towards floor.

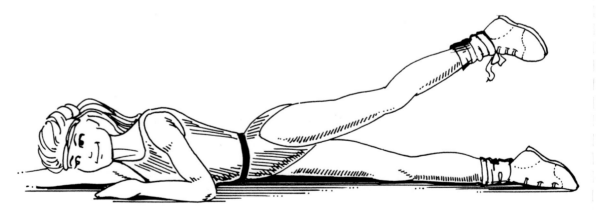

LEG LIFTS AND LEG CIRCLES (Buttocks)

ACTION: Place your knees and elbows on the floor. Keeping
your back straight, lift one leg up and down slowly.
Perform leg circles in both directions and vary the size of the circle.
TIPS: Do not arch the back. (Pull the abdominals in towards the spine.)
Relax the head and neck. Leg lifts and circles should be performed
slowly, with control.
VARIATION: Lift leg with knee bent at 90 degrees.
VARIATION: Alternate bringing the top leg (bent or straight)
to the inside and outside of the bottom leg.

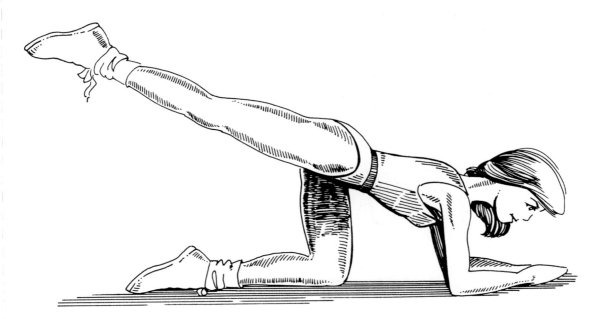

TIGHTENING TIPS:

Remember to repeat all exercises on both sides.
Vary your exercise performance tempo.
There is a tendency in leg work to roll back at the hip and let the powerful
quadriceps (front of the thigh muscles) do the work—watch your
technique.
It is not necessary to lift the legs high for results.
Combine full range of motion exercises with "pulse" movements—take the
leg to the top end of the range and perform small "pulse" movements.

INNER THIGH

PERFORM 15 TO 30 REPETITIONS OF EACH EXERCISE

INNER THIGH LIFTS—KNEE DOWN
ACTION: Lie on side with head supported by bent arm or resting on straight arm. Bring top leg over extended bottom leg and relax top knee into the floor. Lift lower leg up and down.
TIPS: Concentrate on lifting with bottom heel.

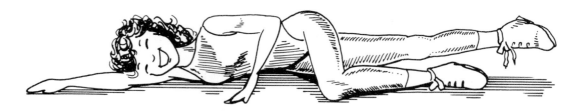

INNER THIGH LIFTS—KNEE UP
ACTION: Same as above. Place top leg over bottom leg with foot in front of knee. Lift lower leg up and down.
TIPS: Concentrate on lifting with the bottom heel.

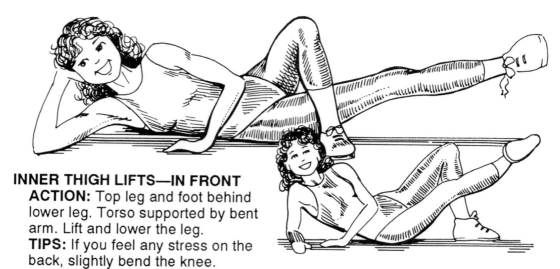

INNER THIGH LIFTS—IN FRONT
ACTION: Top leg and foot behind lower leg. Torso supported by bent arm. Lift and lower the leg.
TIPS: If you feel any stress on the back, slightly bend the knee.
VARIATION: Take the straight leg to the top end of the exercise and perform a small "pulse" movement.
VARIATION: Perform circles in both directions with straight leg.

INNER THIGH SQUEEZES

ACTION: Lie on back with hands under buttocks to tilt pelvis and flatten the spine. Start with knees out and heels together. Press heels together as you extend the legs straight up. Continue pressing heels together as you return to starting position.

TIPS: Perform action with control and keep constant pressure throughout the full range of motion.

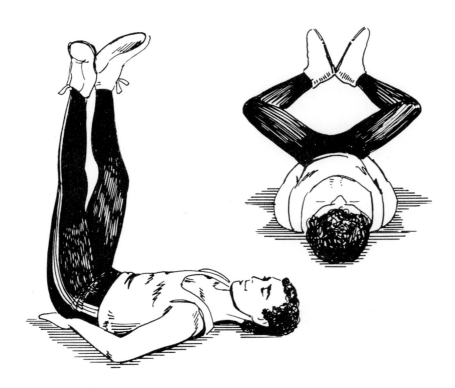

THIGH THOUGHTS TO STRIVE FOR:

Keep the lifting foot parallel to the floor.
Focus on lifting the heel, not the leg.
Remember to perform exercises on both sides.

SUPER SCULPTURING WITH WEIGHTS

If you really want to attain that sleek, firm, and shapely look, use weights. You can work all the major muscles of the body with hand weights.

Perform eight to 20 repetitions of each exercise, doing two to four sets of each before moving to the next. Be sure to rest 30 to 60 seconds between sets.

SQUAT (Buttocks and thighs)
  ACTION: Stand with feet placed wider than shoulders.
  Hold weights into chest or next to shoulders. Keeping your back straight, bend legs and squat down with your buttocks no lower than your knee level and return to start.
  TIPS: Make sure your buttocks go back as you sit and your knees stay over your toes. Do this carefully if you have knee problems!
  VARIATION: Change the width of your stance to work all the muscles completely.

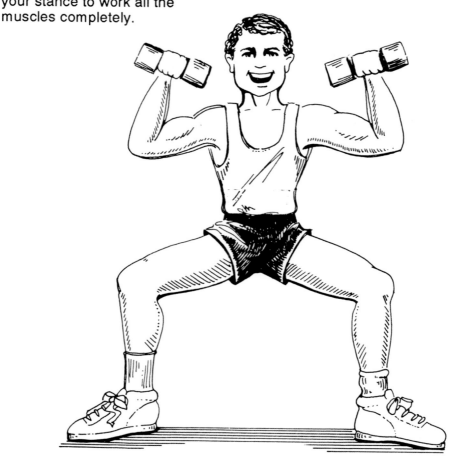

LONG LUNGE (Thighs and buttocks)

ACTION: Stand with feet together and hand weights next to shoulder or down by your side. Step forward about two to three feet with one leg to a bent knee position. Keep the back leg extended, allowing it to bend slightly. Push back to a stand and repeat on other leg.

TIPS: Keep your back straight and press into the bending leg.

VARIATION: Stand with feet together and hand weights by side. "Step back" into lunge position.

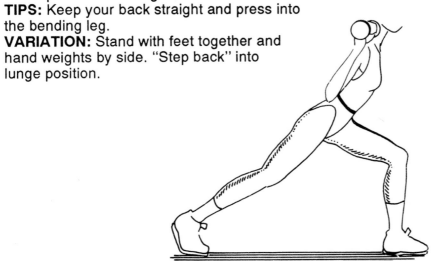

SHORT LUNGE (Thighs and buttocks)

ACTION: Stand with one foot two to three feet in front of the other foot. Hold weights next to your sides. Bend both legs so the back knee comes within six inches from the ground and then straighten up. Do on both sides.

TIPS: Turn toes out slightly for balance.

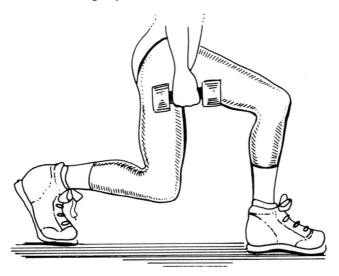

CALF RAISES (Calves)

ACTION: Stand with legs wider than shoulder-width, feet slightly turned out. Hold weights along sides. Lift heels high off the ground and then lower.

TIPS: Perform this exercise on a thick book or block of wood to allow a larger range of motion.

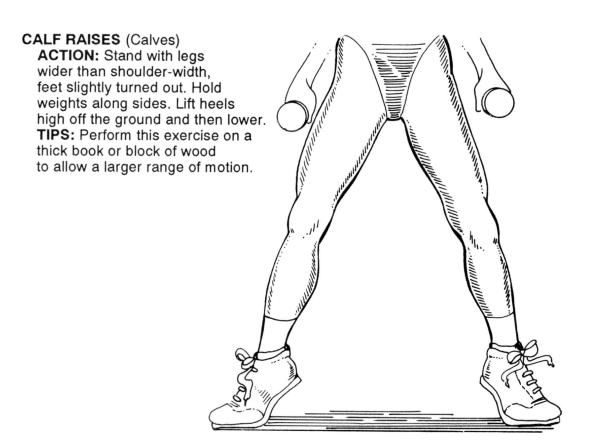

CHEST PRESS (Chest, shoulders, and arms)

ACTION: Lie on a bench or floor with hand weights held by shoulders. Extend arms straight up and back down to side.

TIPS: Keep elbows out from body at the start for effective chest overload. Bend knees with feet on the bench (ground) or with knees pulled towards the chest to safeguard the lower back.

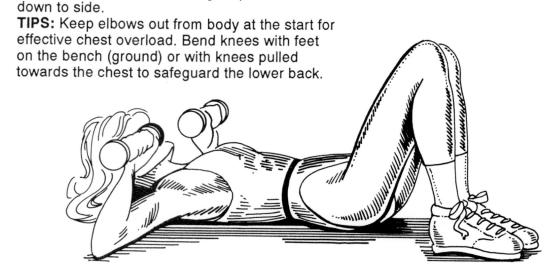

FLYS (Chest and arms)
   ACTION: Same position as chest press. Start with hand weights extended above chest and lower arms perpendicularly away from body and then back up.
   TIPS: Keep arms slightly bent throughout the exercise and palms facing each other.
   VARIATION: Modify the position of the hand weights as they extend over the chest.

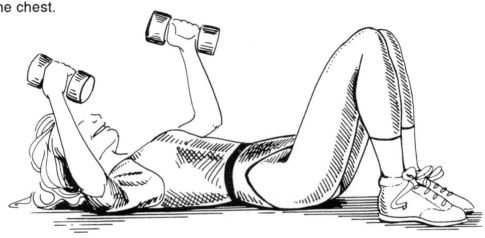

CRUNCHES WITH WEIGHTS (Abdominals)
   ACTION: With back on the floor, weight(s) held behind the head or on the chest, lift upper back off the floor and lower. Lower legs placed on a chair.
   TIPS: Press the small of the back into the floor.
   VARIATION: Twist side to side in the crunch.

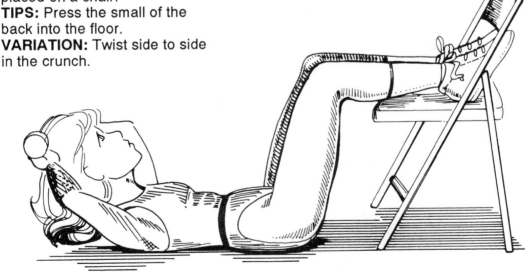

STANDING ROWS (Upper and middle back)

ACTION: Stand in a squatting position with head up, and upper body slightly forward. Hand weights are extended in front of body. Pull elbows as far back as they will go and return to start.

TIPS: Do not bend forward too much (this may stress the spine).

VARIATION: Stand in lunge position with weight in one hand. Bend over at waist and place other hand on bent knee for support. Pull arm straight back and lower.

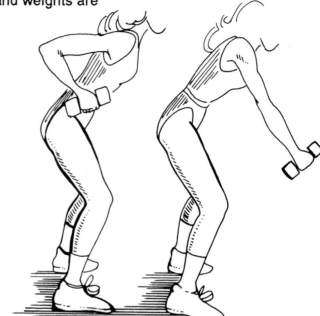

SHOULDER/LATISSIMUS DORSI (Shoulders and latissimus dorsi—side of torso)

ACTION: May be done standing or sitting.

SHOULDER: Start with hand weights held next to shoulder. Press weights straight over head.

LATISSIMUS DORSI: Slowly lower arms bending the elbows. Keep arms out to side and away from the body. Bring the elbows towards the back of torso. Repeat sequence.

TIPS: For effective "lat" work, concentrate on squeezing the elbows into the torso.

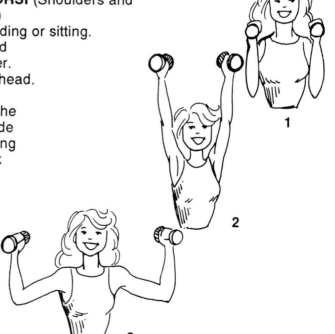

SIDE LATERAL RAISES (Shoulders and back)
   ACTION: Hold hand weights next to your side. Keeping arms
slightly bent, elevate weights laterally to shoulder height and lower.
   TIPS: Do not "lock" elbow joints or raise arms above shoulders.
   VARIATION: For more upper back work, sit in a chair and bend forward
at hips. Lift weights to shoulder height with bent arms and lower.

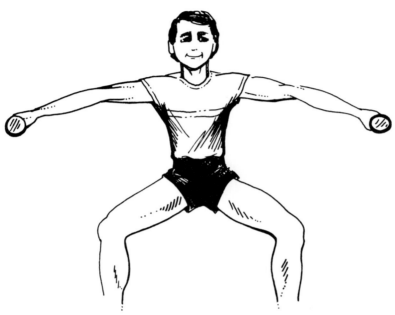

TRICEP EXTENSIONS (Triceps—back of arms)
   ACTION: Stand with legs shoulder-width apart
and knees bent. Bring weights up, bending
elbows up and back. From this position, extend
arms straight back and then return to start.
   TIPS: Keep the elbows from swinging
forward and back.
   VARIATION: Extend elbows to the side
and open arms to the side
(no higher than shoulders).

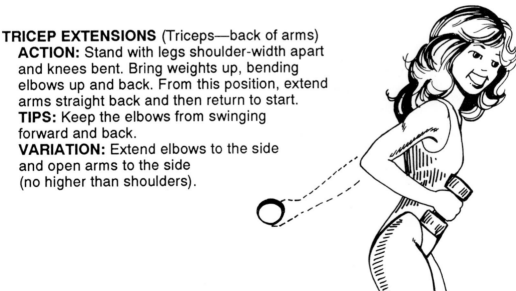

BICEP CURLS (Biceps—front of arms)
    ACTION: Stand with legs shoulder-width apart and knees bent. Bring weights to shoulder and lower.
    TIPS: Keep the hands in a "palm-up" position.
    VARIATION: Alternate lifting one arm and then the other. Or do the curls in a lunge position.

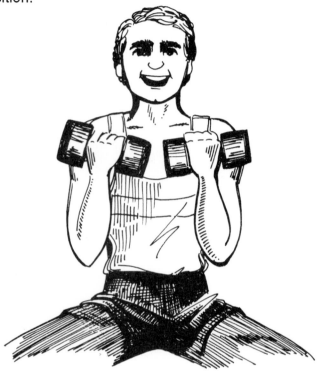

SUPER SCULPTURE SUGGESTIONS:

Find a hand weight that's comfortable, yet challenging.
For variety, vary the number of repetitions, the sequence of exercises, the number of sets, or the weight.
For best results perform this routine two or (preferably) three times a week.
As the weight gets easy to work with, gradually overload with: a heavier weight, more repetitions, more sets, or less time between sets.
Try a circuit training format (time effective and good for muscular endurance training): perform a set of each exercise and then move to the next exercise without resting. Perform two to four circuits.
Refer to A CIRCUIT WORKOUT for more on circuit training.

Try the following circuit training workout for some variety. You can do this workout with and without weights and can add an aerobic station between exercises for a more complete workout.

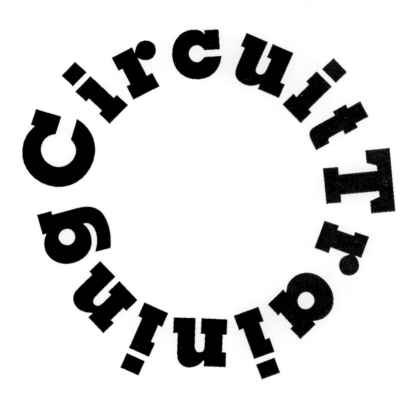

A CIRCUIT WORKOUT

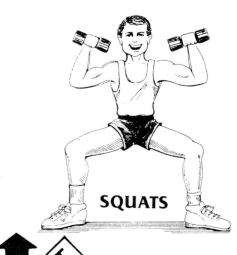

SQUATS

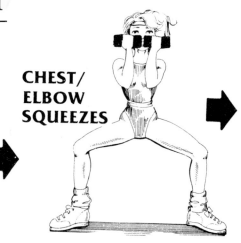

CHEST/ ELBOW SQUEEZES

START

FINISH

Circuit training is one of the most popular forms of training because you constantly move and change from one exercise to another. No rest is needed between exercises since you are working different muscle groups at each station. Circuit training can be performed with or without weights. By placing an aerobic station between each exercise (except for those done lying on the floor), you can burn additional calories and improve your level of fitness.

WIDE-ARMED PUSH-UPS

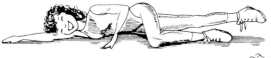

INNER THIGH LIFTS

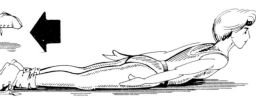

BACK EXTENSIONS

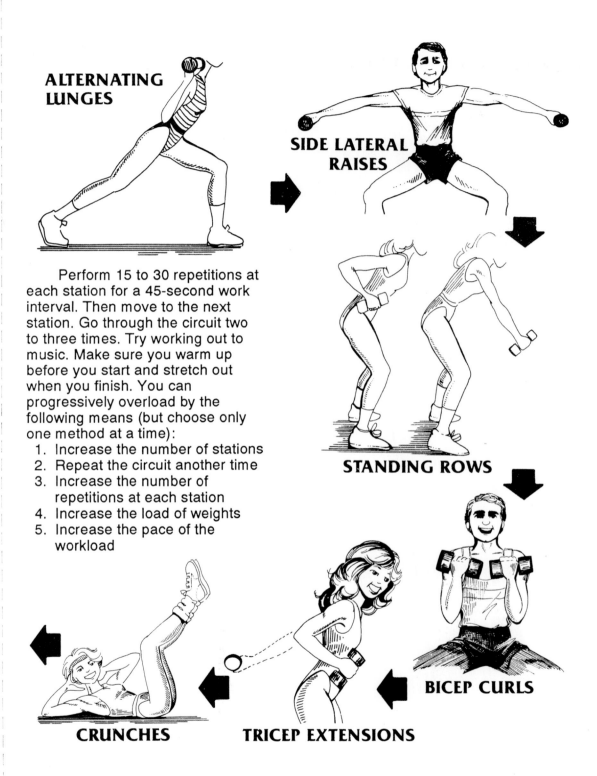

ALTERNATING LUNGES

SIDE LATERAL RAISES

STANDING ROWS

BICEP CURLS

CRUNCHES

TRICEP EXTENSIONS

Perform 15 to 30 repetitions at each station for a 45-second work interval. Then move to the next station. Go through the circuit two to three times. Try working out to music. Make sure you warm up before you start and stretch out when you finish. You can progressively overload by the following means (but choose only one method at a time):

1. Increase the number of stations
2. Repeat the circuit another time
3. Increase the number of repetitions at each station
4. Increase the load of weights
5. Increase the pace of the workload

STRETCH RIGHT!

A well-designed flexibility program focuses on all the muscle groups and joints of the body—not just the most frequently used body parts. Stretch properly to achieve maximum flexibility.

STRETCHING STRATEGY:

Stretch warm muscles, not cold ones.
Avoid bouncing (ballistic) movement. Stretch gradually into and out of the stretch.
Stretch to the point of limitation, not to the point of pain.
Concentrate on relaxing the muscles being stretched; slow breathing helps.
Stretches to improve flexibility should be held 30 to 60 seconds.
Always stretch opposing muscle groups.
Keep the muscles warm when stretching by wearing warm-ups or sweats.
Stretch daily and certainly after every workout.
Increases in flexibility take time; you must be patient.

NECK
ACTION: Very slow circular movement of head towards each shoulder and chest.
TIPS: It is not recommended to take your head back too far—you may possibly stress your neck.

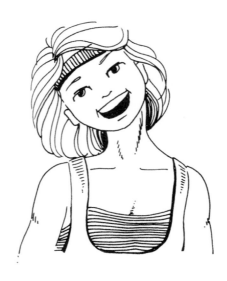

SHOULDERS (two stretches)

1) ACTION: Holding a towel or rope over your head, stretch the arms back.

2) ACTION: Sit on the knees with the front of the feet flat on the floor. With towel behind back, bring the chest to the knees as you stretch the arms away from the body.

TIPS: This is also a very good stretch for the spine and the front of the lower leg!

VARIATION: Change the width of your grip on the towel.

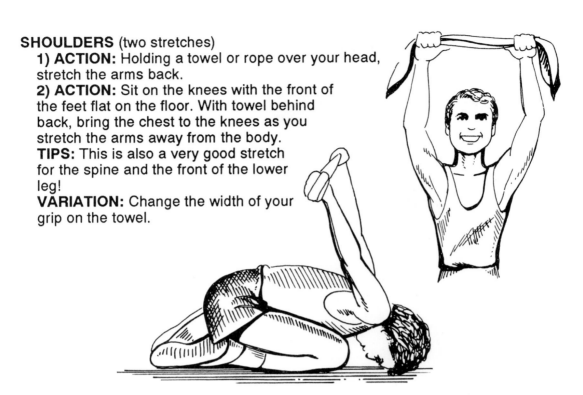

HIPS, SIDE, AND BACK

ACTION: While sitting, bring one leg over other leg. Keep the bottom leg extended (but relaxed at the knee). Rotate the torso to both sides by pushing against floor with hands.

TIPS: Look behind you and think "tall."

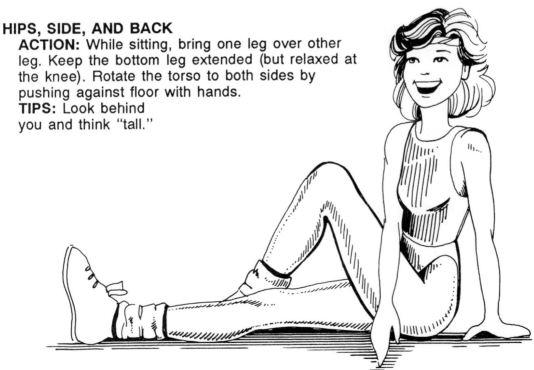

LOWER BACK

ACTION: While lying on the back, grab behind the knees and pull legs towards chest. May be done with legs tucked or slightly extended, but not locked.

TIPS: This also stretches the hamstrings.

VARIATION: This stretch can be performed in the seated position.

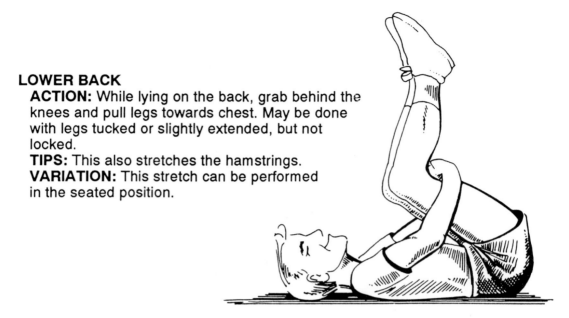

ABDOMINALS AND CHEST

ACTION: From a prone position, lift the shoulders and chest off the ground and support the upper torso with elbows or extended arms.

TIPS: Reach up and out with the upper body.

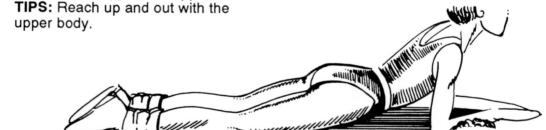

SEATED BUTTERFLY STRETCH (For inner thigh)

ACTION: Bring both heels together and into body. Press knees towards the floor.

TIPS: Grab your ankles, not your toes. Stretch torso forward as well.

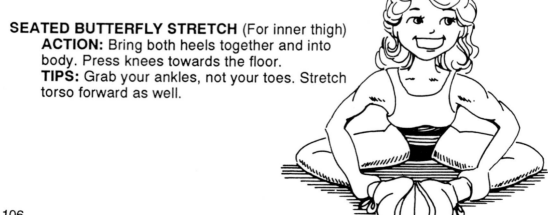

HALF-STRADDLE STRETCH (For hamstrings and lower back)

ACTION: With one leg straight and the other leg bent, reach your chest forward towards the straight leg and hold. Do both legs.

TIPS: Keep the back straight and relax.

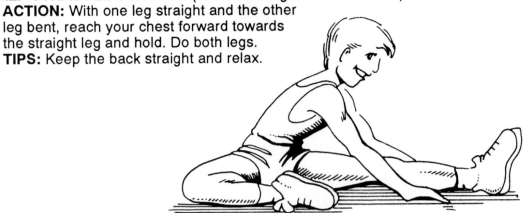

STRADDLE STRETCH (For hamstrings, inner thigh, and lower back)

ACTION: Stretch forward with your upper body between your open legs.

TIPS: Keep your knees facing up, legs straight, and back straight. (Placing your hands on the floor behind your thighs is a good modification for those a little less flexible in this position.)

QUADRICEPS AND HIP FLEXORS

ACTION: While lying on your side, grab below the knee and stretch the leg back.

TIPS: Focus on bringing the leg back and not out to the side.

VARIATION: Do the stretch standing against a wall, next to a chair, or in the prone position.

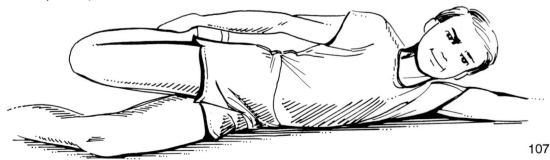

ACHILLES STRETCH AND CALF STRETCH

ACTION: Stand in a lunge position with toes facing forward. To stretch the calf, bend front leg and keep back leg straight. To stretch Achilles tendon (and soleus), bend the back knee keeping the heel on the floor.

TIPS: Sometimes it is best to do these against the wall or an immovable object.

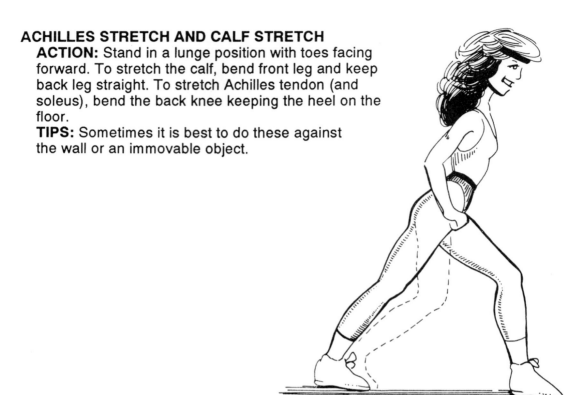

FITNESS FACTS
AND FICTION

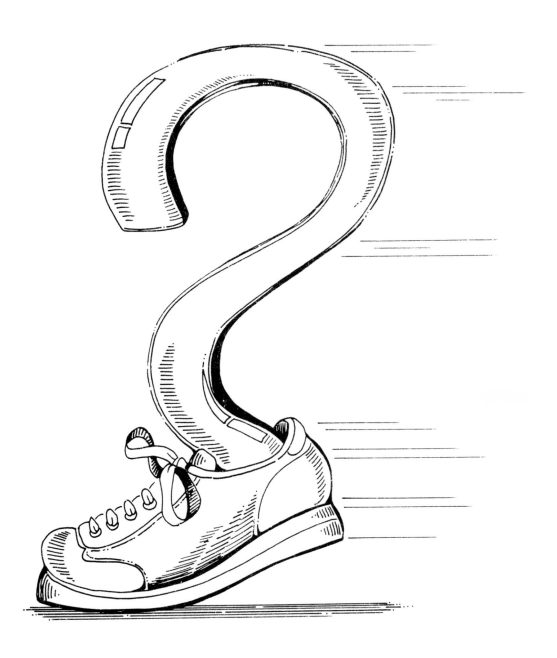

QUESTIONS AND ANSWERS

1) **What are three major factors which contribute to improved health?** Regular aerobic exercise, improved dietary habits, and a positive mental attitude.

2) **How do age and sex affect coronary heart disease risk?** Generally, the older you are, the greater your risk for heart attack. Between the ages of 35 and 44, coronary heart disease is less frequent in women than men, probably due to the production of the female hormone estrogen. Heart attacks appear to even out with older age.

3) **What are the three most important coronary heart disease risk factors?** Cigarette smoking, high blood pressure, and abnormal levels of cholesterol. The risk of heart attack is five times as great if these three factors are present.

4) **Should you exercise on hot, humid days?** Keep it light. Sweat will not evaporate well (to cool you off) in the humidity and you may overheat.

5) **Are "sugary" exercise drinks beneficial during and after exercise?** No, **water** is the best fluid replacement. Sugar can **retard** your absorption of water.

6) **So is it O.K. to drink water while exercising?** Yes, your body's circulation system must get food and nutrients to the working cells. As you sweat and lose water your heart has to work harder. Quench your thirst but don't overdrink!

7) **Should additional salt be taken after exercise?** There's plenty of salt from the food we eat and what we sprinkle on it. Excess salt can irritate the stomach, dry out body tissue, and raise blood pressure.

8) **Do vitamins enhance performance and give energy?** A **surplus** of vitamins probably won't improve your performance. Vitamins don't contain energy, food does, but vitamins **do** help metabolize food.

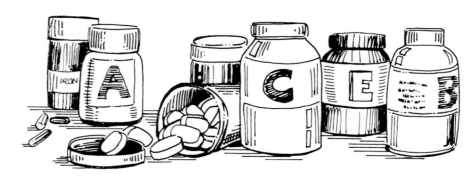

9) **Will I get more out of my workout by speeding up the exercises?** No, smooth, controlled movements, properly executed through the full range of motion at an even tempo are more important than speed.

10) **Do all exercise programs give the same benefits?** No, but everyone needs **sustained,** full-body, vigorous, aerobic activity.

11) **What training effects happen to your body with aerobic exercise?** 1. Your lungs will be able to process more oxygen. 2. The heart becomes a stronger muscle and pumps out more blood with each beat (stroke volume), which in turn allows you to increase oxygen delivery. 3. The blood vessels offer less resistance to blood flow, reducing the work of the heart. 4. The working muscles become more efficient at utilizing oxygen and nutrients for energy (ATP).

12) **What is the difference between saturated and unsaturated fats?** Saturated fats come predominantly from animals and are a suspected contributor to coronary heart disease. Unsaturated fats come from vegetables and are much better for your system.

13) **Can you reduce the number of fat cells in your body?** No, only the size of the fat cells, not their numbers.

14) **What is the fastest way to lose weight?** Weight management is a balance of energy intake (food) and energy output (aerobic exercise). The most efficient method for reducing "fat" weight is to do more aerobic exercise and eat less food.

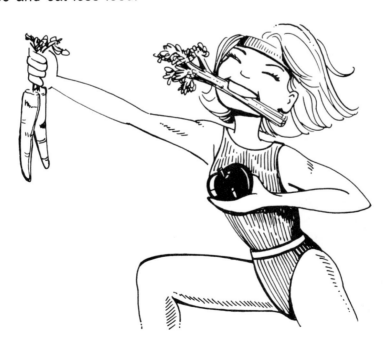

15) **Can you lose weight by diet alone?** Certainly, only you lose a lot of muscle tissue as well as fat. You need exercise, too!

16) **What is the recommended percentage of fat for men and women?** From 12 percent to 18 percent for a man and from 16 percent to 25 percent for a woman.

17) **How is the percentage of body fat determined?** Several popular methods include skinfold calipers, underwater weighing, and electrical impedance analysis.

18) **Is there a difference between being overfat and overweight?** Yes, overweight is only concerned with pounds. Overfat is concerned with the muscle/fat relationship. For instance, many professional football players are overweight by the familiar height/weight charts but have a low percentage of body fat (under 14 percent) and are certainly not overfat.

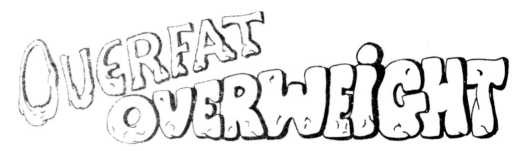

19) **What is your Basal Metabolic Rate (BMR)?** It is the minimal energy requirements of the body at rest. It can be simply estimated by multiplying your body weight in pounds by a factor of 10 or 11 for women and men, respectively. For example, the basal metabolic rate of a 120 pound female is (120 x 10) 1200 Calories per 24 hours.

20) **What happens to your BMR as you age?** Your BMR decreases with age primarily for two reasons. 1. There is often a loss of lean body tissue (muscle) with aging. 2. There is usually a decrease in activity while diet remains constant. This is all the more reason to keep exercising throughout your life!

21) **What are the best foods to eat after aerobic exercise?** A selection of foods rich in complex carbohydrates (starches, not sugars) such as whole grain breads and cereals, pastas, potatoes, leafy vegetables, green beans, broccoli, rice, peas, fruit and grains. But give your body about an hour to recover first!

22) **Will exercise make you tired?** Only temporarily; exercise will ultimately give you **more** energy.

23) **Will exercise enhance your sex life?** You bet! Increased energy, more vitality, higher self-esteem, stress control, and body firmness all contribute to a person's sex life. Right?

24) **How long does it take to realize the benefits of a regular exercise program?** It takes about four to 12 weeks for benefits to appear and up to six months for you to get "hooked" on exercise.

25) **How many days of exercise can you miss before beginning to lose what you've gained?** No more than three days in a row.

26) **How long can you completely layoff exercise before you lose it all?** From five to eight weeks.

27) **What is muscle soreness and how do you get rid of it?** The delayed soreness that appears several hours after exercise (usually 12 to 24 hours) and lasts for 2 to 4 days may be related to actual minute tears in muscle tissue or tears in connective tissue near the muscle or joint. It may also be from muscle spasms or an increase in fluid retention stimulating the pain nerve endings around the joint site. Strange as it seems, performing the same activity that causes muscle soreness will help relieve it. Slow stretching also relieves muscle soreness. Drink plenty of water to enhance the healing process.

28) **What is that pain in the side sometimes felt in aerobics?** That sharp pain below the rib cage, often called a "stitch in the side," is usually caused by poor circulation in the muscles of the diaphragm or rib cage. Slow down your pace to allow the proper dilation of the affected blood capillaries and the pain will go away.

29) **Will exercise give you a longer life?** The aging process cannot be reversed, but exercise may slow down normal physiological deterioration. More importantly, exercise can improve the quality of your life.

30) **What qualities do people who have lived to be 100 have in common?** Moderation and a positive outlook on life. Few smoke and few are fat. They usually get up early and go to bed early. Many claim to have always kept busy during their lives and describe themselves as hard workers. They all seem to be very self-sufficient and protect themselves from too much stress.

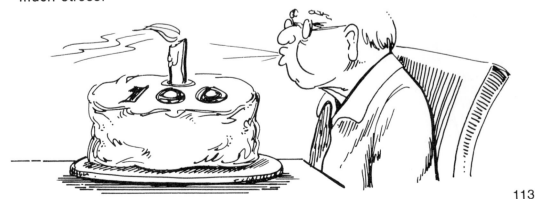

31) **How does smoking affect exercise?** Smoking constricts the bronchial tubes which are the pathways by which oxygen and other gases enter the body. Also the carbon monoxide in cigarette smoke can combine with hemoglobin in red blood cells taking space which should be used to transport oxygen to the exercising muscles. Thus, your cardiorespiratory system must work harder to do the same amount of work.

32) **What is cross-training?** Cross-training is a method of integrating different fitness activities with the purpose of gaining or maintaining total-body fitness while reducing injuries. Each person must find the best mix of aerobics, resistance training, swimming, cycling, racquet sports, walking and recreational sports. It is a very safe, effective, and balanced approach to fitness. Cross-training is extremely effective in a weight loss program as total work and hence caloric expenditure can be increased without increasing the risk of overuse injuries.

33) **What is dietary fiber?** It is basically a type of complex carbohydrate made up of plant material that cannot be digested by the human body. Refining and processing foods removes almost all of the natural fiber. The main sources of dietary fiber are whole-grain cereals and breads, fruits, and vegetables. Optimal amounts of fiber in the diet increase gastric motility and therefore may reduce the incidence of diverticulitis, colon and rectum cancer, and obesity.

34) **Explain what steady-state and anaerobic threshold mean?** Steady-state in aerobic exercise represents a balance between the oxygen needs of the working muscles and their oxygen supply. As exercise intensity increases, the oxygen supply to the working muscles can not meet all the oxygen needs of the muscles and therefore the anaerobic energy systems will contribute more to the total energy production of the working muscles. The eventual transition from predominantly aerobic, oxidative energy production to predominantly anaerobic energy production during increasing exercise intensity is called the anaerobic threshold.

35) **Is there any evidence that exercise can reduce heart disease?** Yes, a scientific study of over 16,000 Harvard alumni suggests that people who expend 2,000 calories per week in brisk exercise reduce death rates from heart disease 25 to 33 percent compared to those who do not exercise. Death rates decreased with increased weekly calorie expenditure up to 3,500 calories, after which there was no advantage to those who did more exercise.

36) **In a typical dance-exercise class consisting of 20 to 30 minutes of aerobic exercise, will loss of excess body fat be maximized at a lower or higher exercise intensity?** Although it is true that exercising at a lower intensity burns predominantly fat and at a higher intensity predominantly carbohydrates, at the higher intensity total caloric expenditure will be greater. Therefore a person should exercise at a higher exercise intensity that can be **safely** maintained for the exercise period if loss of excess body fat is the primary goal of the exercise program.

FAMOUS EXERCISE MYTHS

Myth #1) IF YOU ARE THIN, YOU'RE FIT.
Sorry, but being thin is no indication of how
efficient your heart, lungs and muscles are.
Body composition testing has demonstrated that
many thin people actually have more than the
recommended percentage of body fat. You've
got to exercise!

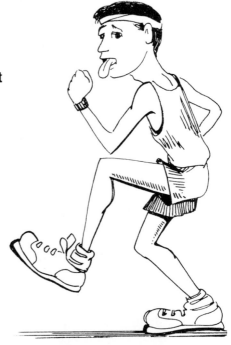

Myth #2) SIT-UPS GET RID OF STOMACH FAT. Wouldn't that be nice!
This myth is based on **SPOT REDUCING.** Research clearly shows that
exercises for specific body areas firm the muscles, but fat reduction comes
from aerobic exercise and a decrease in caloric intake. Fat is reduced
proportionally throughout the body.

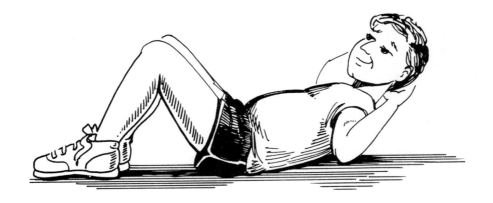

Myth #3) WEIGHT LIFTING DEVELOPS A STRONG HEART. Lifting weights does elevate the heart rate, but this type of exercise does not improve aerobic capacity. It does develop firmer and shapelier bodies.

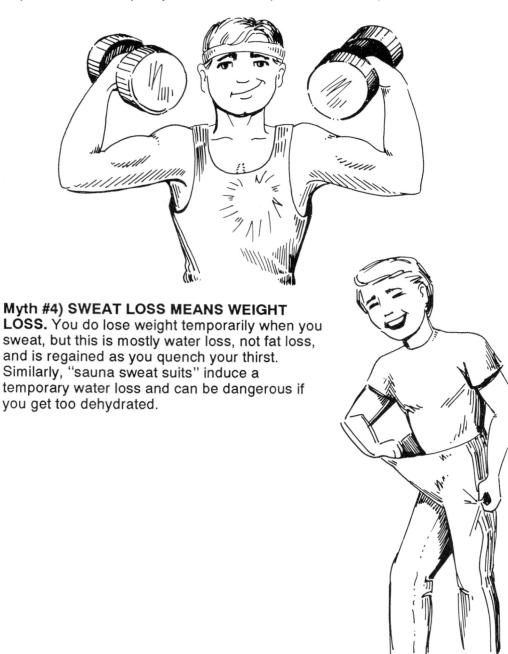

Myth #4) SWEAT LOSS MEANS WEIGHT LOSS. You do lose weight temporarily when you sweat, but this is mostly water loss, not fat loss, and is regained as you quench your thirst. Similarly, "sauna sweat suits" induce a temporary water loss and can be dangerous if you get too dehydrated.

Myth #5) AEROBIC EXERCISE AND JOGGING CAUSE A WOMAN'S BREASTS TO SAG. There is no evidence documenting this claim. However, a good supportive bra is recommended for comfort.

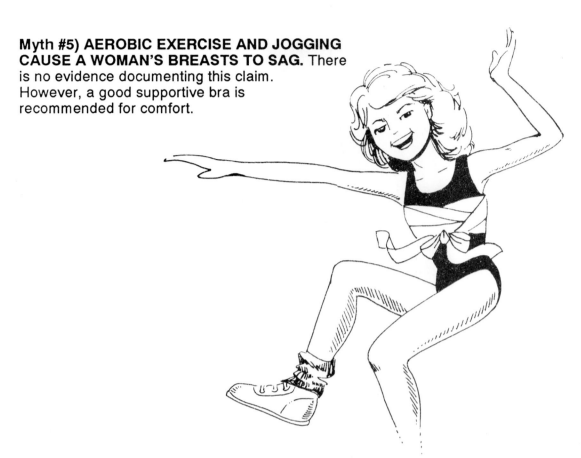

Myth #6) EXTRA PROTEIN MAKES YOU STRONGER. Wouldn't it be great if there really were super foods? If you eat a well-balanced diet, you should consume enough protein for your body's needs. Excess protein is only converted into and stored as fat.

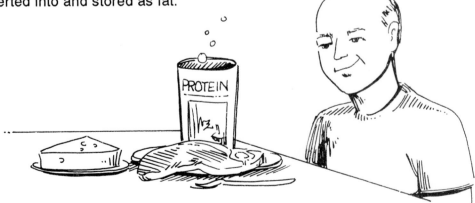

Myth #7) A CANDY BAR (SUGAR) BEFORE EXERCISE WILL GIVE YOU FAST ENERGY. Actually, candy bars, honey, and other sweets quickly enter the bloodstream and stimulate a tremendous release of insulin. The extra insulin during exercise causes your blood sugar to drop, leading to faster exhaustion.

Myth #8) GO FOR THE BURN. Listen to your body. Any type of pain is a warning signal. None of the physiological mechanisms associated with "the burn" have been demonstrated to have beneficial results for you.

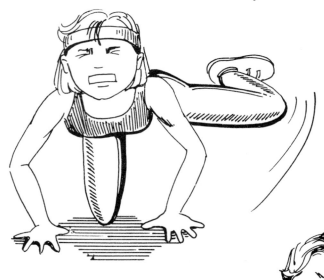

Myth #9) LIFTING WEIGHTS GIVES WOMEN BULKY MUSCLES. Women do not produce enough male hormones to allow for large muscle growth. And women don't have as much muscle fiber or mass as a man. Lifting weights will help a woman develop a better figure.

Myth #10) A LOW RESTING HEART RATE MEANS YOU'RE FIT. Exercise can lower your resting heart rate. However, this alone does not indicate a person's fitness level.

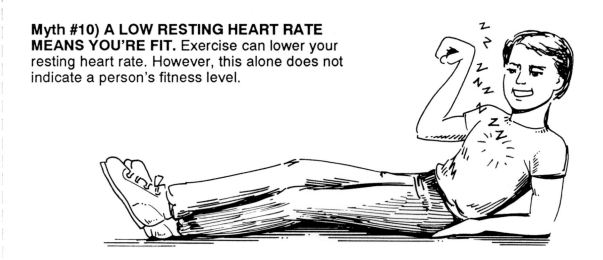

Myth #11) ELECTRICAL STIMULATION CAN REDUCE FAT, INCREASE TONE, AND BUILD STRENGTH. Wow, all those results for just sitting there with electrodes attached to you. How appealing! Though electrical stimulation devices are used by physical therapists for rehabilitation purposes, they are quite ineffective as an effortless exercise alternative.

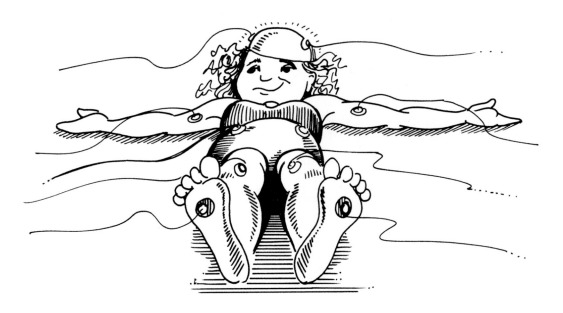

Myth #12) MUSCLES TURN TO FAT WHEN YOU STOP EXERCISING. There are many retired athletes who seem to prove this. However, fat cannot change to muscle (or vice versa). When you stop exercising, your muscles start to waste away and lose their firmness. If you continue to eat a substantial diet (as many of these athletes do), the overconsumption of food will result in larger fat cells.

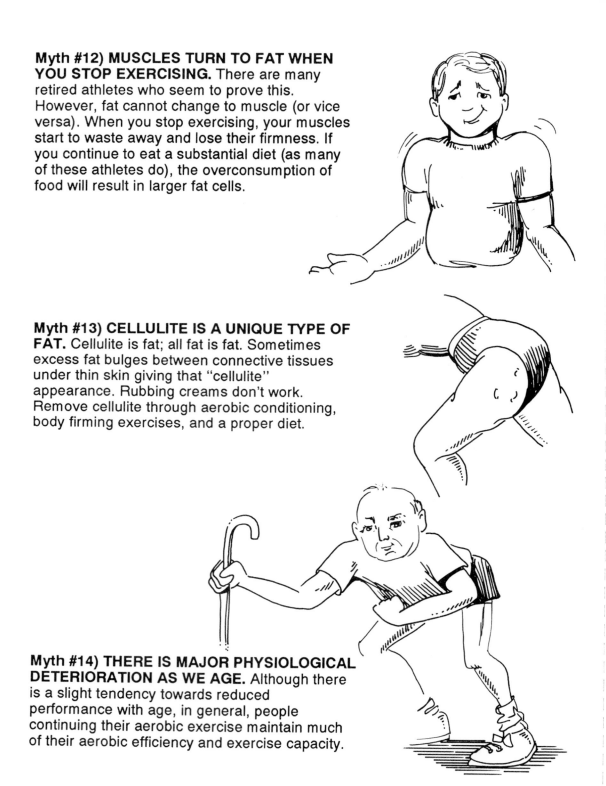

Myth #13) CELLULITE IS A UNIQUE TYPE OF FAT. Cellulite is fat; all fat is fat. Sometimes excess fat bulges between connective tissues under thin skin giving that "cellulite" appearance. Rubbing creams don't work. Remove cellulite through aerobic conditioning, body firming exercises, and a proper diet.

Myth #14) THERE IS MAJOR PHYSIOLOGICAL DETERIORATION AS WE AGE. Although there is a slight tendency towards reduced performance with age, in general, people continuing their aerobic exercise maintain much of their aerobic efficiency and exercise capacity.

FITNESS TRIVIA QUIZ

Try this trivia quiz to learn some additional fitness facts!

1) True or False: The average foot walks more than a thousand miles a year.
2) Is it training **affect** or training **effect**?
3) True or False: Muscles waste away if they are not used.
4) What percent of your body is water? 50%, 60%, 70%.
5) True or False: There are over 600 muscles in the human body.
6) What unique dynamic ability do muscles possess?
7) Which is the single most important source of fuel for your body? Fats, carbohydrates, proteins.
8) What is the junction of two bones called?
9) What is the term for enlargement of muscles?
10) True or False: Before the age of four you have about one half of the number of fat cells you will have as an adult.
11) One pound of fat equals how many calories?
12) The average heart beats how many times a minute? 62, 72, 82.
13) Name four of the six classifications of nutrients you need to eat.
14) True or False: Vitamins contain calories.
15) True or False: Vitamins are named as alphabet letters because, when they were discovered, scientists did not know their chemical structure and could not give them "proper" names.
16) Lack of what mineral is associated with "tired blood?"
17) True or False: Your appetite increases in cold weather.
18) Fast-twitch muscle fiber, known for its explosive characteristics, is referred to as _____ muscle fiber. (red or white)
19) What is the longest muscle in the body?
20) What is the largest tendon in your body?
21) Your skeleton comprises what percent of your body weight? 15%, 25%, 35%
22) How many years does it take for the cell structure of your skeleton to completely rejuvenate itself? 5 years, 7 years, 10 years.
23) True or False: Two-thirds of exercise-induced injuries are caused by overuse.
24) Which is the only joint in the body with 360 degrees of rotation?
25) True or False: Sweat is your body's way of cooling off.
26) What is the single most preventable cause of death?
27) True or False: You burn fewer calories in cold weather than in moderate or warm weather.
28) True or False: Current estimates in the U.S. indicate that about 50% of all adults have a weight problem.
29) How many glasses of water should you drink each day?
30) True or False: Drinking cool water during exercise is beneficial as it reduces internal body heat.

ANSWERS TO FITNESS TRIVIA QUIZ

1) True
2) Training Effect
3) True
4) 70%
5) True
6) They contract
7) Carbohydrates
8) A joint
9) Hypertrophy
10) True
11) 3500 calories
12) 72
13) Carbohydrates, fats, proteins, water, vitamins, minerals
14) False—vitamins do not contain calories
15) True
16) Iron
17) True
18) White
19) Sartorius on the thigh
20) Achilles tendon
21) 15%
22) 10 years
23) True
24) Shoulder
25) True
26) Cigarette smoking
27) False—your body burns more calories in cold weather to stay warm
28) True
29) 8 to 10 glasses
30) True

HOW DID YOU DO?

26 or more correct   You are Exceptional!!!
21 to 25 correct   You can be Proud!!
16 to 20 correct   You should Try Harder!!!
15 or less correct   You are Not Alone!!!

HEALTH AND FITNESS TERMS

ADENOSINE TRIPHOSPHATE (ATP): The high energy substance found in cells from which the body gets its energy.

AEROBIC EXERCISE: Physical activities such as brisk walking, running, cycling, swimming, rowing, and aerobic dancing, that rely heavily upon oxygen for energy production.

ANAEROBIC EXERCISE: "Without oxygen" present; short-term output of energy for muscular contraction when the oxygen supply is insufficient.

ATHEROSCLEROSIS: A slow, progressive disease involving the narrowing of blood vessels, usually arteries.

BALLISTIC: Fast, bouncy movement.

BLOOD PRESSURE: The force that blood exerts against the walls of the blood vessels and that makes the blood flow through the circulatory system.

BLOOD SUGAR: The concentrations of sugar (called glucose) in the blood.

CALORIE: A unit of measure for the rate of heat or energy production in the body.

CARBOHYDRATES: Foodstuffs primarily used for vigorous muscular activity. Found in the body as glucose and glycogen.

CARDIORESPIRATORY ENDURANCE: The capacity of your heart, blood vessels, and lungs to function optimally during sustained vigorous exercise.

CARTILAGE: The resilient covering of the weight-bearing surface of bones. The cartilage absorbs shock and prevents direct wear on the bones.

CHOLESTEROL: A fat-like substance that plays an important role as a building block for cells and hormones. It is obtained from eating foods of animal origin and also produced by the body. Elevated levels are associated with increased risk of heart disease.

CIRCUIT TRAINING: Exercises performed in sequence from station to station. Usually done at a rapid pace.

COOL-DOWN: An "aerobic cool-down" refers to a gradual decrease of vigorous aerobic conditioning. A "workout cool-down" refers to the stretching and relaxation phase at the end of a training session.

CORONARY HEART DISEASE: The impairment of the coronary arteries of the heart associated with a build-up of cholesterol and fatty substances on the inner artery wall.

DEHYDRATION: The condition that results from excessive loss of water.

ENERGY: The capacity or ability to perform work.

EXERCISE HEART RATE: The heart rate during aerobic exercise that will result in cardiorespiratory benefits. Also referred to as "training heart rate."

FAT: A food substance used as an energy source. It is stored when excess fat, carbohydrate, or protein is ingested.

FLEXIBILITY: The range of motion of a joint or group of joints.

FREQUENCY: Refers to the number of workouts needed per week to establish a training effect.

GLUCOSE: Energy source (in the form of sugar) transported in the blood.

GLYCOGEN: The form in which glucose is stored in the body (primarily in the liver).

HEART ATTACK: Death of a part of the heart muscle caused by a lack of blood flow.

HEART RATE: The number of times the heart beats per minute.

HYPERTENSION: High blood pressure.

HYPERTROPHY: An increase of mass in a muscle from resistive exercise.

INTENSITY: The level of physiological stress on the body during exercise.

ISOKINETIC CONTRACTION: A contraction in which the tension is constant throughout the range of motion.

ISOMETRIC (STATIC) CONTRACTION: A contraction in which tension is developed but there is no change in the length of the muscle.

ISOTONIC CONTRACTION: A contraction in which the tension varies throughout the range of motion.

LACTIC ACID: The product of incomplete metabolism that can occur when insufficient oxygen is supplied to the active muscle. Believed to be a contributing factor to fatigue.

MAXIMUM HEART RATE: The highest your heart will beat during aerobic exercise.

MAXIMUM OXYGEN CONSUMPTION: The maximal rate at which the muscles can consume oxygen in one minute.

MINERALS: Inorganic substances of the body including sodium, potassium, chloride, calcium, phosphorous, magnesium, sulfur, and at least 14 trace minerals that perform several necessary roles in the body.

MUSCULAR ENDURANCE: The ability to exert force (not necessarily maximal) over an extended period of time.

NUTRIENTS: The basic substances of the body obtained by eating foods.

OBESITY: An above-average amount of fat in the body.

OVERLOAD: To exercise a muscle or group of muscles with resistance greater than normally encountered.

PROTEIN: A food substance that sustains basic structural properties of the cells and serves as a source for hormones and enzymes in the body.

RECOVERY HEART RATE: The gradually declining heart rate following the cessation of aerobic exercise.

REPETITION: A repetition represents each time an exercise movement is completed.

RESTING HEART RATE: The average heart rate prior to initiating any physical activity.

SATURATED FAT: Animal fat and fat found in dairy products and eggs that contribute to atherosclerosis.

SET: Group(s) of repetitions. One set might consist of 10 repetitions.

SKINFOLD: A pinch of skin and subcutaneous fat from which total body fat may be estimated.

SPOT REDUCING: A myth that fat can be specifically reduced from one body area through exercise.

STATIC STRETCH: A stretch which is held.

STRENGTH: The capacity of a muscle to exert force against resistance.

STROKE VOLUME: The amount of blood pumped by the left ventricle of the heart per beat.

VITAMINS: Nutrients required in micro amounts that are essential to numerous bodily functions.

WARM-UP: The first portion of a workout, designed to prepare the body for the vigorous exercise to follow.

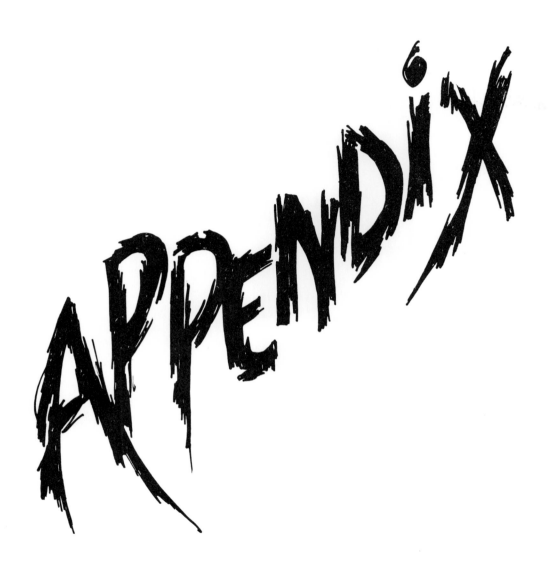

THE MUSCLE SYSTEM

MUSCLE AND EXERCISE CHART

This chart lists the major muscle groups and specific exercises presented in this book, as well as the opposing groups.

Deltoids
Push-up Variations
Dips
Side Laterals
Chest Press

Pectorals
Chest Press
Wide-arm Push-ups
Flys

Rhomboids and Trapezius
Standing Rows

Latissimus Dorsi
Shoulder/Latissimus Dorsi

Biceps
Bicep Curls
Chest/Elbow Squeeze

Triceps
Tricep Extensions
Dips
Pike Push-ups
Chest Press

Abdominals
Crunch Variations

Obliques
Twisting Crunches
All-Around Crunches
Rope Pull Crunches

Spinal Extensors
Back Extensions

Gluteals
Squats
Lunges
Prone Leg Lifts
Leg Lifts and Leg Circles

Quadriceps
Squats
Lunges

Hamstrings
Squats
Lunges

Thigh Adductors
Inner thigh Variations

Thigh Abductors
Outer Leg Lifts
Side Leg Circles
Forward Side Leg Lifts

Gastrocnemius and Soleus
Calf raises

Achilles Tendon
(Connects gastrocnemius to heel)

EXAMPLES OF OPPOSING MUSCLE GROUPS

BICEPS vs. TRICEPS
DELTOIDS vs. LATISSIMUS DORSI
PECTORALS vs. RHOMBOIDS AND TRAPEZIUS
QUADRICEPS vs. HAMSTRINGS
ABDOMINALS vs. SPINAL EXTENSORS
THIGH ABDUCTORS vs. THIGH ADDUCTORS

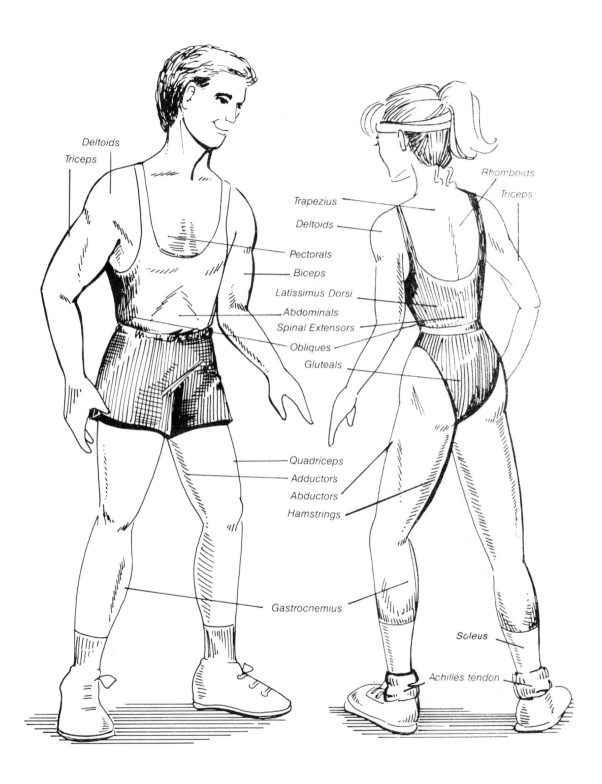

Deltoids
Triceps
Trapezius
Deltoids
Pectorals
Biceps
Latissimus Dorsi
Abdominals
Spinal Extensors
Obliques
Gluteals
Rhomboids
Triceps
Quadriceps
Adductors
Abductors
Hamstrings
Gastrocnemius
Soleus
Achilles tendon

YOUR HEALTH AND FITNESS PROFILE

HEALTH AND FITNESS EVALUATION LIST

What personal health and fitness habits are you happy with? _____

_____
_____
_____
_____
_____
_____
_____
_____

What health and fitness changes would you like to make? _____

_____
_____
_____
_____
_____
_____

What short-term goals (12 weeks away) would you like to achieve? _____

_____
_____
_____
_____
_____
_____

What long-term goals (one year) would you like to achieve? _____

_____
_____
_____
_____
_____
_____
_____

PHYSICAL FITNESS PROFILE

Beginning Date _____   **Retest Date** _____

AEROBIC EFFICIENCY
STEP TEST:

Score _____   Score _____
Rating _____   Rating _____

1.5 MILE RUN:

Score _____   Score _____
Rating _____   Rating _____

ROCKPORT WALKING TEST:

Score _____   Score _____
Rating _____   Rating _____

MUSCULAR STRENGTH AND ENDURANCE
ABDOMINAL CRUNCHES:

Score _____   Score _____
Rating _____   Rating _____

PUSH-UPS: MODIFIED OR STANDARD

Score _____   Score _____
Rating _____   Rating _____

FLEXIBILITY
SIT AND REACH:

Score _____   Score _____
Rating _____   Rating _____

BODY COMPOSITION
BODY FAT TEST:

Score _____   Score _____
Rating _____   Rating _____

PERSONAL DATA
AGE _____ RESTING PULSE _____ WEIGHT _____ TARGET ZONE _____

TARGET BODY WEIGHT

You can estimate your desired body weight by using your percentage of body fat. Follow the example below.

1. Your weight in lbs.		150	lbs.
2. Skinfold body fat measurement result (Round off to whole number)		22	%
3. Fat weight (your weight x item 2)		150 x .22 = 33	lbs.
4. Lean body weight (your weight – item 3)		150 – 33 = 117	lbs.
5. Desired percent body fat		17	%
6. Desired weight (item 4 ÷ (1.00 – item 5)		117 ÷ (1 – .17) = 141	lbs.
7. Pounds to gain or lose (your weight – item 6)		150 – 141 = 9	lbs.

NOW ESTIMATE YOUR DESIRED BODY WEIGHT

1. Your weight in lbs.			lbs.
2. Skinfold body fat measurement result (Round off to whole number)			%
3. Fat weight (your weight x item 2)			lbs.
4. Lean body weight (your weight – item 3)			lbs.
5. Desired percent body fat			%
6. Desired weight (item 4 ÷ (1.00 – item 5)			lbs.
7. Pounds to gain or lose (your weight – item 6)			lbs.

CALORIC EXPENDITURE CHART

You can easily estimate the number of calories you expend during aerobic exercise activities. To determine the number of calories expended, multiply the total number of minutes of activity times the Calories per minute. For example, a 110 pound woman doing 20 minutes of continuous aerobic dance would expend approximately 172 Calories (8.6 x 20 = 172).

CALORIC EXPENDITURE CHART
FOR SELECTED AEROBIC ACTIVITIES

(Aerobic dance, cycling, brisk walking, rope skipping, rowing on a machine, running, skating, and swimming)

Your weight in pounds	95 to 104	105 to 114	115 to 124	125 to 134	135 to 144	145 to 154	155 to 164	165 to 174	175 to 184	185 to 194	195 to 204
Calories per minute	8	8.6	9.0	9.7	10.3	11	11.5	12	12.7	13.3	13.7

Values may vary from individual to individual.

_____

_____

Total number of minutes of aerobic exercise _____

Calories expended per minute according to your weight _____

Your estimated caloric expenditure _____

LOOK ALIVE! Workout Chart

1. Go for it!	2.	3.	4.	5.
6.	7.	8.	9.	10.
11.	12.	13.	14.	15.
16.	17.	18.	19.	20.
21.	22.	23.	24.	25. Keep Pushing!
26.	27.	28.	29.	30.
31.	32.	33.	34.	35.
36.	37.	38.	39.	40.
41.	42.	43.	44.	45.
46.	47.	48.	49.	50. Fantastic!

Record the date of each day's workout.

POWER SCULPTURING EXERCISES

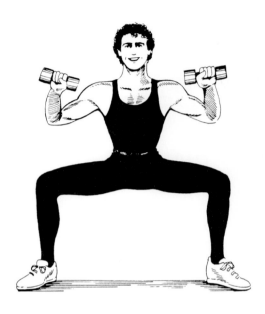

A SPECIAL SUPPLEMENT TO
ANYBODY'S GUIDE TO TOTAL FITNESS

The following "power" exercises are new movement combinations biomechanically designed to effectively challenge the body. This program will offer creativity, movement selection, and exercise sequence to your conditioning program. Begin with a comfortable starting weight and gradually overload with heavier resistance. For variety, perform the standing power exercises in random order changing movements after every eight repetitions. Do all movements with control.

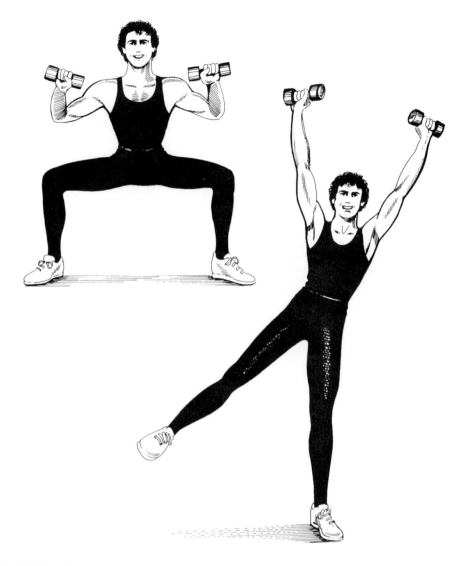

POWER SIDE (Abductors, adductors, gluteals, quadriceps, hamstrings, deltoids, triceps)

ACTION: From a wide squat, extend legs lifting one leg off the ground as you straighten your arms. Return to squat and alternate sides.
TIPS: Keep the lifting leg from rotating outward in order to effectively work the abductors. On all squats, be sure to keep the buttocks at or above standing knee height.

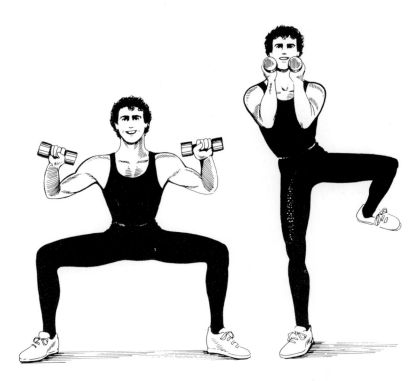

POWER SKI (Abductors, adductors, gluteals, quadriceps, hamstrings, deltoids, pectorals)

ACTION: From a wide squat, extend legs and lift and flex one leg as you squeeze your elbows together. Return to wide squat and alternate sides.
TIPS: Make sure you lift your knee to the side. Keep legs slightly wider than shoulder width in all wide squats.

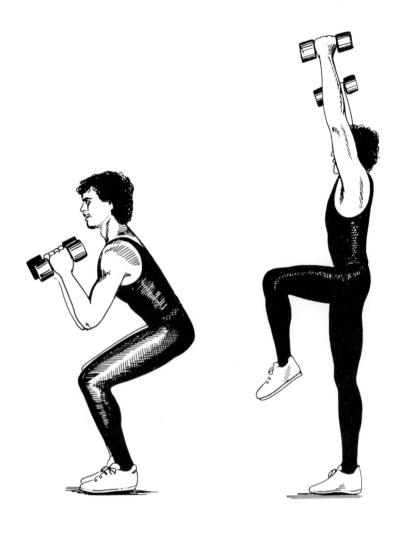

POWER KNEE (Quadriceps, gluteals, hip flexors, deltoids, triceps)

ACTION: From a narrow squat position with legs close together, extend legs lifting one leg with a bent knee as you extend the arms over the head. Lower to narrow squat and alternate sides.

TIPS: Keep your back straight and the buttocks back as you sit in a narrow squat. Do not go as low in the narrow squat as you do in the wide squat.

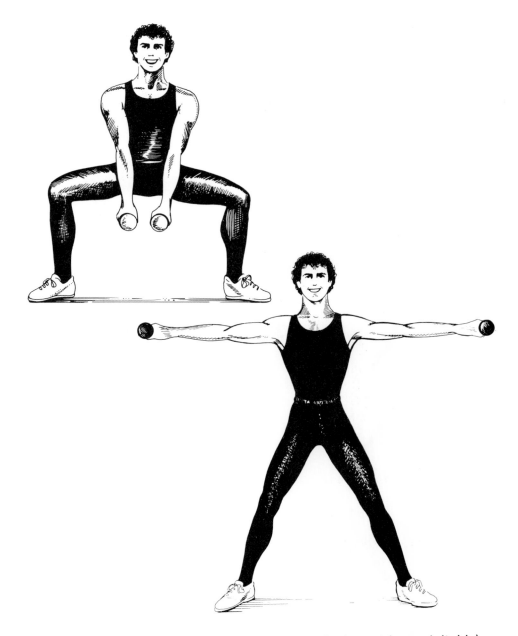

POWER DELTOID (Adductors, quadriceps, gluteals, hamstrings, deltoids)

ACTION: Extend your legs from a squat as you laterally raise your arms to shoulder height. Lower and repeat.

TIPS: Raise and lower your arms (with control) making sure to keep them shoulder height or below in the top position.

139

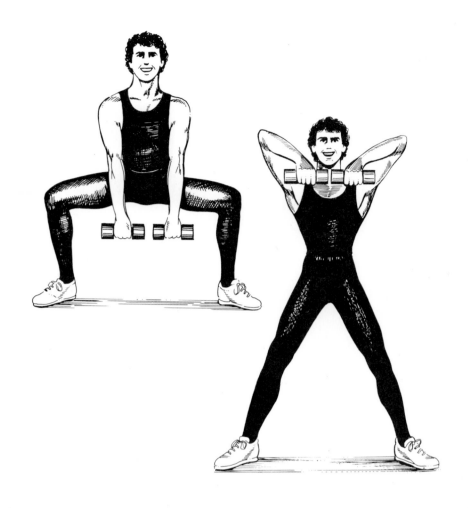

POWER ROW (Spinal extensors, quadriceps, gluteals, hamstrings, trapezius)

ACTION: Extend your body and legs from a flexed squat position as you lift your elbows above your head.

TIPS: Keep your hands close together, stopping them under your chin at the top position. In order to effectively work the spinal extensors, you need to find a comfortable yet challenging starting position where the trunk is flexed. Keep the head up and the back straight.

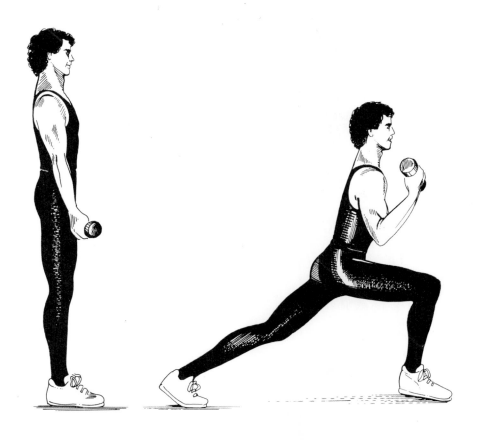

POWER LUNGE (Quadriceps, hamstrings, gluteals, biceps)

ACTION: From a standing position with arms by your side, step back into a lunge position and perform a bicep curl with your arms. Return to the starting position and repeat on other side.
TIPS: Be sure to keep your bent knee over your ankle and your weight forward.
VARIATIONS: Turn your knuckles toward your shoulders and perform a reverse arm curl. You can also vary the degree of difficulty by keeping your knees slightly bent throughout the exercise.

POWER SCULPTURE SEQUENCE

Here is a recommended sequence of exercises for your muscular endurance training taken from this supplement and *Anybody's Guide to Total Fitness.* You will effectively work your body's muscular system progressing from larger (more energy demanding) muscle groups to smaller (more specific) muscles. To overload, vary the number of repetitions, the number of sets, the movement tempo, or the weight. Perform exercises half-time using music with 140–150 beats per minute.

Standing Power Moves: Power side, power ski, power knee, power row, power deltoid, power lunge.

Gastrocnemius/Anterior Tibialis: Calf raises with feet facing out, forward, and in. Toe lifts for anterior tibialis.

Pectorals: Standing flys with bent arms (arms high and low), chest/elbow squeezes.

Rhomboids/Trapezius: Standing row, single arm row, reverse fly (standing or with one knee on the floor).

Abdominals: Crunch, twisting crunch, rope pull crunch, all-around crunch, reverse crunch (all abdominal exercises with or without hand weights).

Specific Gluteals, Abductors, Adductors: Prone leg lifts, outer leg lifts, inner thigh lifts.

Deltoid/latissimus dorsi: Shoulder/latissimus dorsi (in seated position).

Triceps/deltoid/chest: Wide-arm push-ups, pike push-ups, triceps extension on knees (or seated).

Biceps: Single arm bicep curls (in seated position).